NEUROSCIENCE RESEARCH PROGRESS

HYDROCEPHALUS

SYMPTOMS, TREATMENT AND POTENTIAL COMPLICATIONS

Neuroscience Research Progress

Additional books in this series can be found on Nova's website under the Series tab.

Additional E-books in this series can be found on Nova's website under the E-book tab.

Neurology - Laboratory and Clinical Research Developments

Additional books in this series can be found on Nova's website under the Series tab.

Additional E-books in this series can be found on Nova's website under the E-book tab.

NEUROSCIENCE RESEARCH PROGRESS

HYDROCEPHALUS

SYMPTOMS, TREATMENT AND POTENTIAL COMPLICATIONS

AMAYA VELAZQUEZ
EDITOR

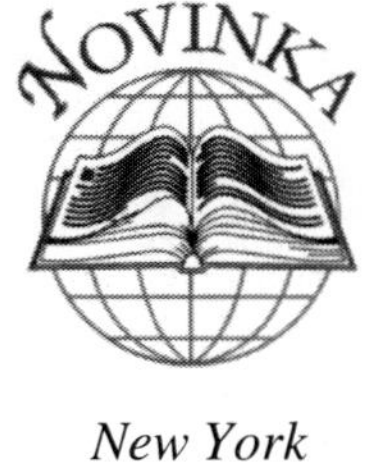

New York

For permission to use material from this book please contact us:
Telephone 631-231-7269; Fax 631-231-8175
Web Site: http://www.novapublishers.com

Library of Congress Cataloging-in-Publication Data

Library of Congress Control Number: 2012955261
ISBN: 978-1-62417-725-5

Published by Nova Science Publishers, Inc. † New York

CONTENTS

PREFACE

Hydrocephalus as a clinical entity is usually defined as the presence of an excess amount of water (CSF, cerebrospinal fluid) resulting in increased pressure inside the head with variable clinico-pathological implications. In this book, the authors discuss the symptoms, treatment and potential complications of hydrocephalus. Topics include the features and management of hydrocephalus; normal-pressure hydrocephalus as a common source of elderly incontinence with brain etiology; pediatric hydrocephalus; and hemorrhagic hydrocephalus.

Chapter 1 - Hydrocephalus is a multifaceted clinical entity with multiple etiological factors resulting in the altered state of CSF dynamics, protean clinical manifestations, varied neuro-radiological presentations and multitudes of available treatment strategies for satisfactory palliation but as yet no one full proof risk free curative treatment available. Basically, there is disturbance of one or more of the normal physiological mechanisms involved in the production, circulation and absorption of the CSF. There is a plethora of classifications and terminologies to clinically define it.

However, the each designated term defines its one or more aspects well but some other aspects largely remain unaccountable or unexpressed and therefore, such terms are mainly semantic and remain short of their objectives.

It is commonest in the early age group with complex issues (3-4 cases per 1000 live births): fetal-neonatal-infantile period associated with intracranial hemorrhages and congenital malformations in significant number of cases.

In other pediatric age groups, it is fairly common with and without congenital malformations, obstructive pathologies for the CSF circulation including congenital problems, acquired CNS infections and hemorrhages as well as developing neoplastic conditions. Trauma remains a rare cause of hydrocephalus.

The symptoms and signs are combinations of increased volume of the head or the CSF containing intracranial spaces as compared to the normal subjects as well as increased intracranial pressure and their combined deleterious effects on the anatomy (brain parenchyma and intracranial spaces) and physiology of the brain (cerebral irritation phenomena, developmental delays, as well as imminent or progressive raised intracranial pressure effects).

In young adults and middle ages, the etiology of the hydrocephalus is usually simple and more straight forward, and in a great majority of cases it is mainly due to obstructive pathologies(tumors, infections, trauma, hemorrhage, etc) affecting the ventricular system or subarachnoid spaces. These patients are commonly present with tetrad of clinical symptomatology: headaches, vomiting, visual obscuration and papilledema.

Interestingly in the elderly, there lies a great challenge to prove the entity and then to find its etiology. However in the literature, there is some proof to say and support the concept that intermittently, there is a mild increase in the intracranial pressure with or without ventricular enlargement and associated cerebral atrophy as a main culprit for the triad of its symptoms (ataxia, dementia and incontinence).

Following clinical evaluation, irrespective of age, then the initial assessment is performed with variable combinations of ultrasound of the head, the CT scans of the head and spine, and the MRI scans of the cranio-spinal region. The laboratory results are needed where indicated as in cases of meningitis, brain hemorrhage, etc.

Patient's clinical status, neuro-imaging findings and parents' perceptions are main determinants of the further management of these cases.

Management comprises mainly the clinical observations in the border line cases. However, the medical therapy is advised for the mild degrees of hydrocephalus and the surgical therapy remains gold standard treatment for the patients with moderate to severe grades of proven hydrocephalus where raised ICP is well demonstrated and the patient is likely to be benefitting with the operative interventions mainly for the diversion of the CSF under increased pressure. The surgical procedures are not without risks mainly such as hemorrhage, infection, obstruction, shunt failures, etc. Considerable morbidities and mortality still exist despite remarkable advancement in the neuro-radiological procedures(Modern Ultrasound procedures, CT Head, MRI scans), improvement in surgical procedures with cautions and care, modern anesthetic techniques and sophisticated post operative care and the periodic

OPD follow ups. There are many surgical methods but currently ventricular-peritoneal shunt and third ventriculostomy are in vogue being associated with lower rates of morbidities and mortality.

Untreated patients have extremely poor prognosis with large head, thin cerebral parenchyma, and moribund clinical state and largely generate great anxiety and frustration in parents on one side and medical faculty on the other.

Chapter 2 - The symptoms of hydrocephalus are developed by the increased intracranial pressure. The main symptoms observed among children include poor feeding, excessive sleepiness, enlarging head with soft areas on the fontanelles, an inability to move eyes upward, and vomiting. Commonly observed symptoms among adults include headache, nausea, ataxia, and visual disturbances. Generally, the earliest and most prominent symptoms of hydrocephalus are balance and gait disturbances. Furthermore, impairment of memory and urgency incontinence is common.

The goal of the treatment for hydrocephalus is to protect the periventricular tissues from pressure and osmotic loads. In order to do so, the intracranial pressure needs to be reduced by decreasing the cerebrospinal fluid (CSF) volume. The medical treatment is decreasing CSF secretion by the choroid plexus-acetazolamide and furosemide and increasing CSF reabsorption-isosorbide. However, surgical CSF diversion is mostly performed. Among the surgical interventions, ventriculoperitoneal (VP) shunt is most commonly used, and, recently, neuroendoscopic techniques are utilized to treat obstructive hydrocephalus.

Hydrocephalus can cause some complications, or complications may develop as a result of the surgery used to treat it. The potential complications of hydrocephalus include cerebral atrophy, neurological deficits, cerebral ischemia, and dementia. The complications of shunt are malfunctions, blockages, and infections.

Chapter 3 - This chapter reviewed a common source of elderly incontinence with brain etiology, normal-pressure hydrocephalus (NPH), from auro-neurological point of view. This disease manifests with gait disturbance, dementia, and urinary incontinence as a clinical triad. Urinary frequency/ urgency (overactive bladder) often precedes urinary incontinence in this disease, and in some patients may be the early manifestation. While NPHis less common than white matter disease in the elderly, at approximately one-tenth the prevalence, it is particularly important because the symptoms can be reversed by shunt surgery or endoscopic third ventriculostomy. Bladder overactivity due to frontal hypofunction, which normally tonically inhibits the micturition reflex, commonly underlies OAB in this disease. Recent brain

SPECT imaging has shown close relationship between frontal hypofunction and OAB, both of which are dynamically improved after shunt surgery in this disease.

Chapter 4 - Hydrocephalus can occur in infancy and it often coexists with many congenital and acquired brain disorders. The diagnosis and management of hydrocephalus present common problems in pediatric patients. Diagnosis of pediatric hydrocephalus often require high index of suspension and early detection with institution of treatment can prove to be pivotal in order to prevent long-term complication. Surgery still remains as mainstream treatment for pediatric hydrocephalus. Various surgical approaches have been advocated, and VP shunt is by far the most commonly practiced procedure worldwide. Patients with implanted VP shunts may present with complex and challenging problems that include infection and obstruction of the shunt.

Therefore insertion of a VP shunt represents a lifetime commitment for the child and family and the decision to treat can be difficult and it should not be taken lightly. Mortality has significantly reduced with modern surgical technique, yet there is still much long-term morbidity associated with the disorder. Multidisciplinary planning and close follow-up is needed to ensure the maximal developmental potential of these children.

In this chapter the authors will discuss the clinical features, diagnosis, and management of pediatric hydrocephalus.

Chapter 5 - Genetic factors play a role in the development of human hydrocephalus. However, little is known about the pathogenesis of human congenital hydrocephalus. Recently, the authors identified coiled-coil domain-containing 85C (*Ccdc85c*) as a causative gene for hemorrhagic hydrocephalus (*hhy*) mouse mutation exhibiting an autosomally recessive pattern of inheritance. Mice homozygous for *hhy* develop communicating hydrocephalus at near-perfect penetrance, with heads bulged from accumulating cerebrospinal fluid within several days after birth. These mice exhibit a variational ventricular dilatation with frequent brain hemorrhage at biopsy and also develop subcortical band heterotopia, a malformation of cerebral cortex in all cases. Furthermore, these mutant mice showed agenesis of the ependymal layer lining the cerebral cortex, a possible cause of hydrocephalus. Analyses of corticogenesis at embryonic days revealed that premature depletion of cortical radial glia, neural progenitors performing both embryonal neurogenesis and postnatal gliogenesis, underlay the *hhy* phenotype. The *hh*y mutant may be a useful animal model in understanding the pathogenesis of hydrocephalus.

In: Hydrocephalus
Editor: Amaya Velazquez

ISBN: 978-1-62100-453-0

Chapter 1

CURRENT CONCEPTS OF HYDROCEPHALUS AND ITS MANAGEMENT

Rewati Raman Sharma,[1,*] Apollina Sharma[2] and Sameer Raniga[3]

[1]National Neurosurgery Centre, Department of Neurosurgery, Khoula Hospital, Muscat, Oman. Khoula Hospital, Muscat, Oman
[2]Department of Accident-Emergency, Khoula Hospital, Muscat, Oman, Kasturba Medical College, Manipal University, Mangalore, Karnataka, India
[3]Khoula Hospital, Muscat, Oman

ABSTRACT

Hydrocephalus as a clinical entity is usually defined as the presence of an excess amount of water (CSF, cerebrospinal fluid) resulting in increased pressure inside the head with variable clinico- pathological implications.

Hydrocephalus is a multifaceted clinical entity with multiple etiological factors resulting in the altered state of CSF dynamics, protean clinical manifestations, varied neuro-radiological presentations and multitudes of available treatment strategies for satisfactory palliation but as yet no one full proof risk free curative treatment available. Basically,

* Tel/Fax: 00 968 24567339, GSM/Cell: 00 968 99241189/99207852, E-mail: drsharma.rr@ gmail.com, rrsharma@omantel.net.om, drrrsharmaneurosurgeon@ yahoo.com.

there is disturbance of one or more of the normal physiological mechanisms involved in the production, circulation and absorption of the CSF. There is a plethora of classifications and terminologies to clinically define it.

However, the each designated term defines its one or more aspects well but some other aspects largely remain unaccountable or unexpressed and therefore, such terms are mainly semantic and remain short of their objectives.

It is commonest in the early age group with complex issues (3-4 cases per 1000 live births): fetal-neonatal-infantile period associated with intracranial hemorrhages and congenital malformations in significant number of cases.

In other pediatric age groups, it is fairly common with and without congenital malformations, obstructive pathologies for the CSF circulation including congenital problems, acquired CNS infections and hemorrhages as well as developing neoplastic conditions. Trauma remains a rare cause of hydrocephalus.

The symptoms and signs are combinations of increased volume of the head or the CSF containing intracranial spaces as compared to the normal subjects as well as increased intracranial pressure and their combined deleterious effects on the anatomy (brain parenchyma and intracranial spaces) and physiology of the brain (cerebral irritation phenomena, developmental delays, as well as imminent or progressive raised intracranial pressure effects).

In young adults and middle ages, the etiology of the hydrocephalus is usually simple and more straight forward, and in a great majority of cases it is mainly due to obstructive pathologies(tumors, infections, trauma, hemorrhage, etc) affecting the ventricular system or subarachnoid spaces. These patients are commonly present with tetrad of clinical symptomatology: headaches, vomiting, visual obscuration and papilledema.

Interestingly in the elderly, there lies a great challenge to prove the entity and then to find its etiology. However in the literature, there is some proof to say and support the concept that intermittently, there is a mild increase in the intracranial pressure with or without ventricular enlargement and associated cerebral atrophy as a main culprit for the triad of its symptoms (ataxia, dementia and incontinence).

Following clinical evaluation, irrespective of age, then the initial assessment is performed with variable combinations of ultrasound of the head, the CT scans of the head and spine, and the MRI scans of the cranio-spinal region. The laboratory results are needed where indicated as in cases of meningitis, brain hemorrhage, etc.

Patient's clinical status, neuro-imaging findings and parents' perceptions are main determinants of the further management of these cases.

Management comprises mainly the clinical observations in the border line cases. However, the medical therapy is advised for the mild degrees of hydrocephalus and the surgical therapy remains gold standard treatment for the patients with moderate to severe grades of proven hydrocephalus where raised ICP is well demonstrated and the patient is likely to be benefitting with the operative interventions mainly for the diversion of the CSF under increased pressure. The surgical procedures are not without risks mainly such as hemorrhage, infection, obstruction, shunt failures, etc. Considerable morbidities and mortality still exist despite remarkable advancement in the neuro-radiological procedures(Modern Ultrasound procedures, CT Head, MRI scans), improvement in surgical procedures with cautions and care, modern anesthetic techniques and sophisticated post operative care and the periodic OPD follow ups. There are many surgical methods but currently ventricular-peritoneal shunt and third ventriculostomy are in vogue being associated with lower rates of morbidities and mortality.

Untreated patients have extremely poor prognosis with large head, thin cerebral parenchyma, and moribund clinical state and largely generate great anxiety and frustration in parents on one side and medical faculty on the other.

Keywords: hydrocephalus, congenital, acquired, fetal, neonatal, infantile, adult, communicating, non-communicating, obstructive, etiology, patho-physiology, management strategies, shunting procedures, endoscopic third ventriculostomy, clinical outcome, morbidities and mortality

INTRODUCTION

Hydrocephalus is a single most important challenging problem in the neurosurgical practices with so far no sight of its curative solution. Only the palliative treatment is as yet possible in great majority of neurosurgical patients with variable outcome and considerable morbidity as well as mortality.

Hydrocephalus is commonest in the neonatal period due to congenital etiological factors including malformations and thereafter, its incidence gradually decreases. In pediatric neurosurgery, about one third of cases comprises of hydrocephalus with or without associated congenital malformations.

However, in adult neurosurgery, it is only about 5 % of the cases who need shunt surgery for the hydrocephalus due to various etiological factors.

Hydrocephalus may present seemingly benign course at one end and life threatening emergencies at the other end of its clinical spectrum and therefore needs periodic/continuous vigilance as per the given clinical case. The clinical presentation and management will vary on case to case basis.

DEFINITIONS

There is plethora of terms used in relation to the hydrocephalus to define the anatomic-clinical entities, its etiologies, clinical effects and direct consequences as well as the implications of its management strategies and outcome.

Basically, there is problem of production, circulation or absorption properties of the CSF at one or more intracranial sites. Therefore, simplistically, the hydrocephalus may be defined as an excess amount of intracranial CSF under increased intracranial pressure with its clinical implications. This is quite true in a great majority of cases.

1. Layman's perception: The term hydrocephalus usually means to a layman as the Head filled with the excess amount of water (Figure 1). At times, the head appears like a watermelon. It gives impression to the parents that they have not achieved a perfect baby with a normal brain and as if some amount of the brain is being replaced with the added amount of water inside the head. The water is under high pressure which causes further damage on the brain cells and thereby, on their functions. It has significant implications on the psycho-motor development of the baby, childhood learning and teenager's behavior, earning skills in adults and even, the casual life in the old ages.
2. General medical perception: The hydrocephalus per se means excess amount of CSF in the cerebral ventricles under high intracranial pressure at the cost of brain tissues and their functions. Here, water (CSF) under high pressure is filling the head. This can be due to many etiological factors. This is in contrast to the patients with benign intracranial hypertension; where, there is increased intracranial pressure with increased brain swelling but no obvious hydrocephalus. Here, the swollen brain matter under high pressure is filling the head. In normal pressure hydrocephalus (NPH), there is mild to moderate dilatation of the ventricles with normal intracranial pressure and no significant cerebral atrophy. In this situation, neither the water under

high pressure is filling the head, nor there any swollen brain under high pressure in the head. Here, the differentiation needs to be made from the arrested hydrocephalus and ex vacuo phenomenon of the cerebral atrophy.

3. Morphological Forms: Morphologically, the hydrocephalus presents differently in different age groups. In great majority of neonates and infants, it presents with the enlargement of the head and simultaneous reduction in the cortical mantle; whereas in adults, there is actually no change in the head size but there is reduction in the size of brain parenchyma and proportionally increase in the CSF containing spaces. Interestingly, in the elderly (NPH), there may not even be any change in their head size, brain matter size and the size of the CSF containing spaces.

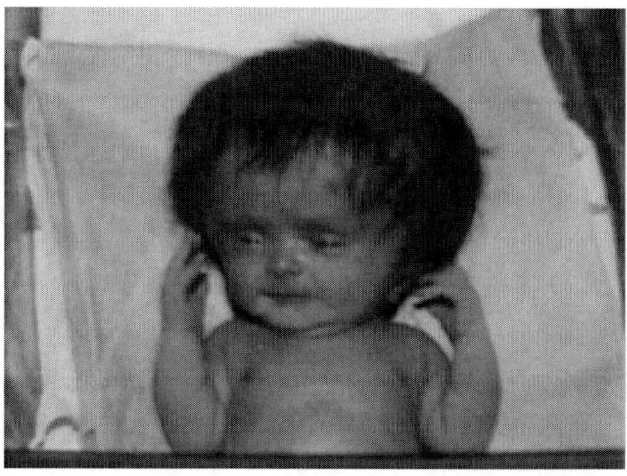

Figure 1. Typical external features with large head in this congenital hydrocephalic baby.

Classification of Hydrocephalus [1-3]

Hydrocephalus is a clinical feature of varied etiological processes but is not a disease entity in itself. Therefore, it is merely semantic to classify hydrocephalus which is one of the many important expressions of various disease processes; although, such classification does offer some help in understanding the overall management of such cases.

1. External versus internal hydrocephalus: [1-3] In external hydrocephalus, there is an abnormal accumulation of the CSF in the basal and superolateral subarachnoid spaces of an infant with nearly normal ventricular system. It is, relatively, a less common and benign condition which gets corrected over a period of time in majority and therefore, periodic ultra-sonographic monitoring is needed. Whereas, the more common condition of internal hydrocephalus is said to occur when there is significant ventricular dilatation along with attenuated subarachnoid spaces. This condition needs prompt management strategy.
2. Congenital versus acquired hydrocephalus: [1-3] Hydrocephalus presents since intrauterine life (prenatal) and the baby is born with it (due to a demonstrable or non-demonstrable cause) is called congenital hydrocephalus {hydrocephalus associated with conditions such as aqueduct stenosis (Figure 2), Dandy- Walker syndrome, Arnold-Chiari malformation, myelodysplasia, etc}. Acquired hydrocephalus occurs due to an etiological factor acquired in post-natal period such as neoplasm, infection, trauma, etc.

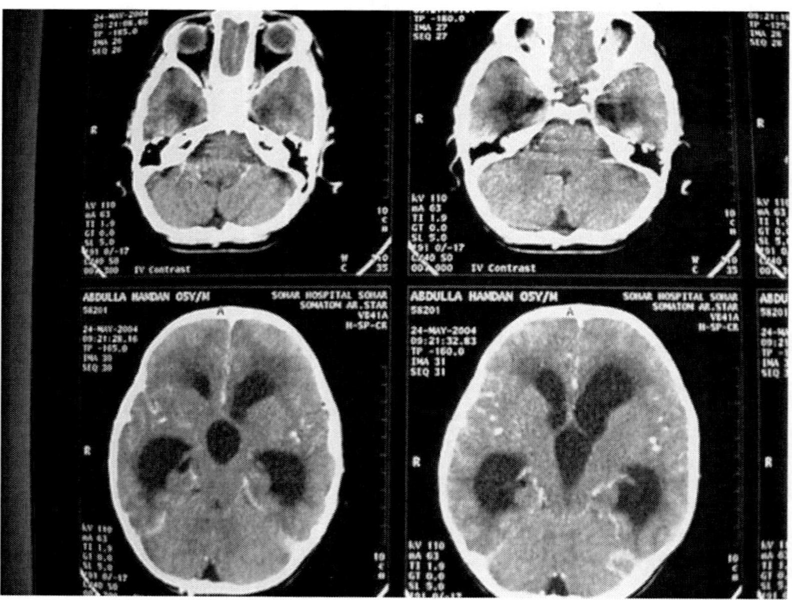

Figure 2. The contrast CT head showing typical tri-ventricular hydrocephalus with normal fourth ventricle in this case of aqueductal stenosis and had ruled out any significant brain stem lesion or posterior fossa tumor.

3. Progressive (active) versus non-progressive (inactive/arrested) hydrocephalus: [1-3]

   a. Progressive hydrocephalus means gradual increase in the ventricular size with increase in the intracranial pressure. Initially there is merely an increase in the ICP without much ventricular dilatation but later the ventricular enlargement becomes obvious on serial US/CT/MRI scans.
   b. Non-progressive hydrocephalus suggests there is an arrest in the progression of the ventricular size with maintenance of normal ICP and resulting in stabilized neurological status. The factors, which were actively responsible for the ventricular dilatation in the past, have become inactive.
      Progressive hydrocephalus needs clinical management and non-progressive hydrocephalus the follow up observations in the outpatient clinic (OPD) as few of these cases may have potential to deteriorate and decompensate in future due to unknown reasons or after mild infection/ trauma.

4. Communicating versus non-communicating hydrocephalus: [1-3] All these clinical cases need proper evaluation and effective medical/surgical management.

Anatomically, it reflects the enlargement of the CSF containing spaces. There is loss of the brain substance mainly with variable increase in the size of the ventricular system, either focally or in general, depending on the site of the obstruction in the pathway of the CSF circulation. When the point of obstruction is in the ventricular system or at its outlets, the hydrocephalus is termed as non-communicating to the subarachnoid spaces. It is termed communicating if ventricular system is in direct communication with the subarachnoid spaces.

A. Communicating hydrocephalus: When ventricular system has no obvious obstructing pathology and all its chambers are communicating freely with each other as well as with the subarachnoid spaces: the obstructing pathology is usually beyond the fourth ventricle outlets, mainly in the basal subarachnoid cisterns, supero-lateral cortical sulci, arachnoid granulations/villi or venous sinuses /superior sagittal sinus. The cause of the communicating hydrocephalus is, mostly, less well appreciated on the neuro-imaging studies.

B. Non-communicating hydrocephalus: depending on the dilatation of the ventricular system

i. Uni-ventricular (obstruction at one foramen of Monro, trapping of the ventricular horns)
ii. Bi- ventricular (obstruction in the anterior third ventricle-like colloid cyst)
iii. Tri- ventricular (obstruction at the posterior third ventricle, aqueduct and posterior fossa)
iv. Tetra- ventricular (obstruction at the fourth ventricular outlets- foramen Magendie and Luschka).

The cause of the non-communicating hydrocephalus is, mostly, very well appreciated on the neuro-imaging studies.

5. ICP-DEPENDANT: [4] Hydrocephalus may be classified based on the ICP readings.

These are two types-

A. High pressure hydrocephalus: The ICP measurements show higher readings most of the time.
B. Normal pressure hydrocephalus: [5] The ICP readings are normal most of the time; except, occasional or periodic increases. This condition typically occurs in elderly patients (Figure 3).

6. TEMPORAL PROFILE: [6-7] When the time course of ventricular enlargement is considered along with the severity of the clinical symptomatology and a relative urgency of the management. A. Acute hydrocephalus means hydrocephalus developing over a short period of time (1-7 days), B. Sub-acute hydrocephalus developing between one to four weeks period (1-4 weeks) and C. Chronic hydrocephalus usually takes more than one month period in its manifestation.

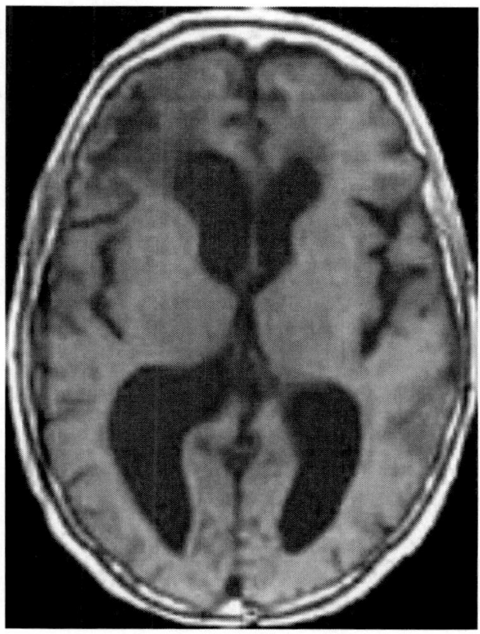

Figure 3. T1 weighted MRI scan showing moderately dilated ventricles with open supero-lateral cortical sulci and sylvian cisterns.

ETIOLOGY OF THE HYDROCEPHALUS [1-3,6-7]

1. Congenital Hydrocephalus

The incidence of congenital hydrocephalus among the new born babies varies in different parts of the world. There are diverse causes of congenital hydrocephalus, although the prematurity and intra-ventricular hemorrhages are the most common ones.

a. Intra-uterine/ fetal hydrocephalus—Periodic antenatal follow ups with ultrasound studies discovered higher incidences of fetal hydrocephalus with some intracranial/neural tube defects [aqueduct stenosis (forking, peri-aqueductal gliosis, intra-luminal septum, etc), Arnold Chiari malformation, Dandy-Walker syndrome (Figures 4 and 5), myelodysplasia (Figure 6), etc] and somatic anomalies. Intrauterine infection, hemorrhage, vascular occlusions, inheritable X-linked aqueduct stenosis, Goldenhar-Gorlin syndrome, ocular malformations, etc are important etiological factors in this period.

Intrauterine infections such as toxoplasmosis, initially, cause ependymitis and then intra-parenchymal peri-vascular granulomas and vascular occlusions as well as aqueduct stenosis with hydrocephalus; and cytomegalovirus initially causes meningo-encephalitis which later results in adhesive arachnoiditis and hydrocephalus. Rarely, congenital hydrocephalus may also be caused by chorio-meningitis virus and group B Coxsackie viruses. These infective conditions need treatment in their own rights along with the hydrocephalus which may need surgical attention. In cases of hydrocephalus due to inheritable X-linked aqueductal stenosis, the CSF shunting usually does not improve their mental retardation. Congenital hydrocephalus (associated with myelomeningocele and type II Arnold Chiari malformation) needs prompt treatment (shunt surgery) as well as the repair of the menigomyelocele at the same time and dealing with the Arnold Chiari malformation at a second stage as and when needed.

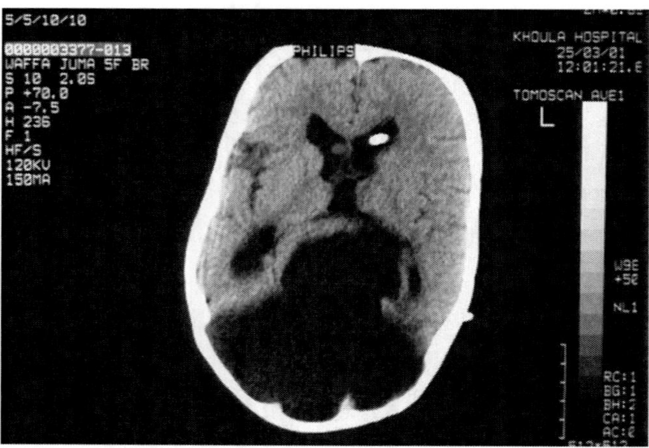

Figure 4. Dandy-walker syndrome with aqueduct stenosis : Supra-tentorial functioning shunt. The patient was admitted for infra-tentorial shunting procedure.

Dandy-Walker malformation (Figures 4 and 5) due to the fourth ventricular outlet block (atresia of the foramina of Magendie and Luschka) resulting in hydrocephalus, large cystic expansion of fourth ventricle, hypoplastic vermis. Shunting of both the lateral and fourth ventricles separately is most rewarding in these cases. Direct excision of the posterior fossa arachnoid cyst presenting with associated triventricular hydrocephalus is needed to relieve the hydrocephalus with or without shunting.

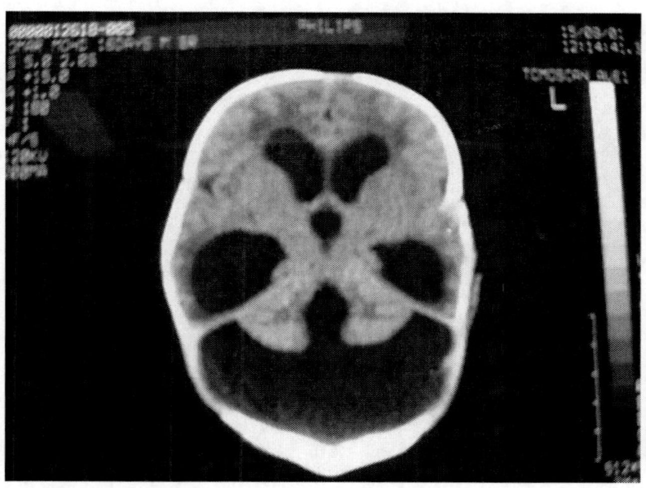

Figure 5. The CT head showing typical features of tetra-ventricular hydrocephalus due to Dandy- Walker syndrome.

2. Acquired Hydrocephalus

A. In pediatric age groups (neonatal, infantile and childhood) :

There are many etiological factors leading to hydrocephalus. Common causes include intra-ventricular hemorrhage associated with prematurity in about 40-50 % of premature babies, bacterial meningitis-ventriculitis, post traumatic hydrocephalus, etc ; less common causes are peri-natal asphyxia and low birth-weight baby and rarely brain tumors may present with hydrocephalus. Even the metabolic causes and metal toxicity may cause transient hydrocephalus. [8-9]

In premature distressed neonatal baby, the intra-cerebral hemorrhage [1-9] occurs mainly in the sub-ependymal germinal matrix of the lateral ventricle. It may subsequently rupture in the lateral ventricle causing blockage either in the intra-ventricular compartment, subarachnoid spaces and or arachnoid granulations and villi.

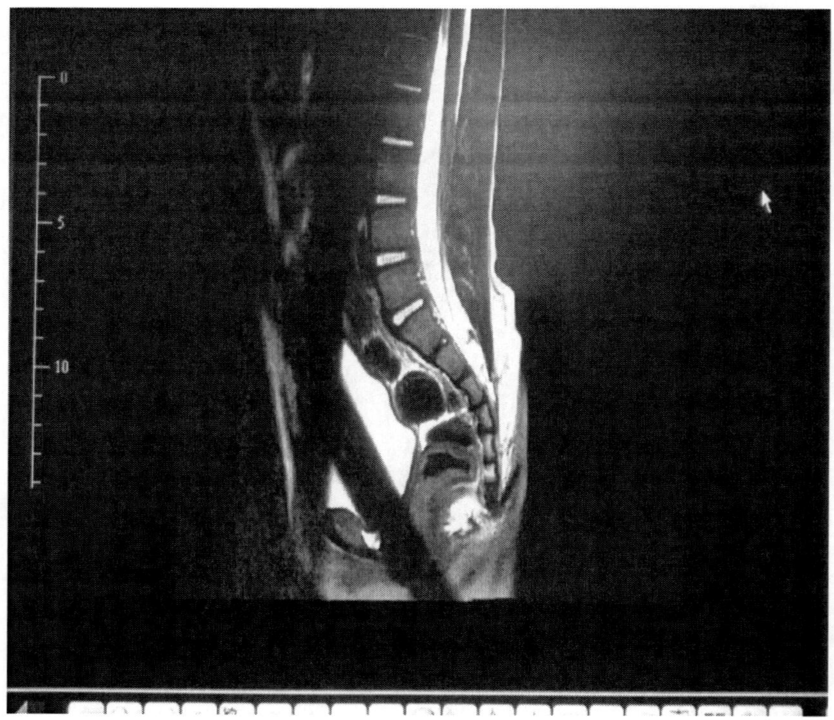

Figure 6. The picture showing low lying conus with tethered spinal cord in a case treated for hydrocephalus.

Consequent hydrocephalus occurs only in about 50% of these cases and is usually of the mild communicating type but less frequently, it may be acute obstructive hydrocephalus due to aqueductal block. Temporizing measures such as serial lumbar punctures in communicating hydrocephalus; whereas, in non-communicating hydrocephalus, ventricular tapping, Ommayya reservoir, and an external ventricular drain are employed although with some risks of infection. A functioning shunt is a difficult preposition in some cases of intraventricular bleeds. But, it must be under taken as soon as possible and feasible using a valveless shunt system with in-line reservoir for flushing/aspirations to minimize the shunt revisions. Interestingly, the infection rate in these shunted babies is about 50% and about 25% of these cases develop ventricular loculations needing more than one shunt with consequent morbidities and mortality. Bacterial meningitis especially due to enteric gram-negative organisms [10] is more common than other organisms in this period and present with severe purulent meningo-ventriculitis and multiloculated/multi-septate compartmentalized hydrocephalus with loss of brain parenchyma (porencephalic cysts). These changes pose a great challenge in their management with shunt surgery, endoscopic lysis of septations, subdural collections and collapse of cortical mantle. These cases are associated with poor development, high morbidities and mortality. Post traumatic hydrocephalus in infancy may present with subdural hematomas and macrocephaly. [11-12] There are clinical problems related to three variables-hydrocephalus, subdural hematomas and a large head (Figure 7). These are treated with valve regulated programmable shunts for the ventricular system and a valveless system for the subdural collections. Once clinically stabilize then the reduction cranioplasty may be considered with attendant risks of morbidities and mortality.

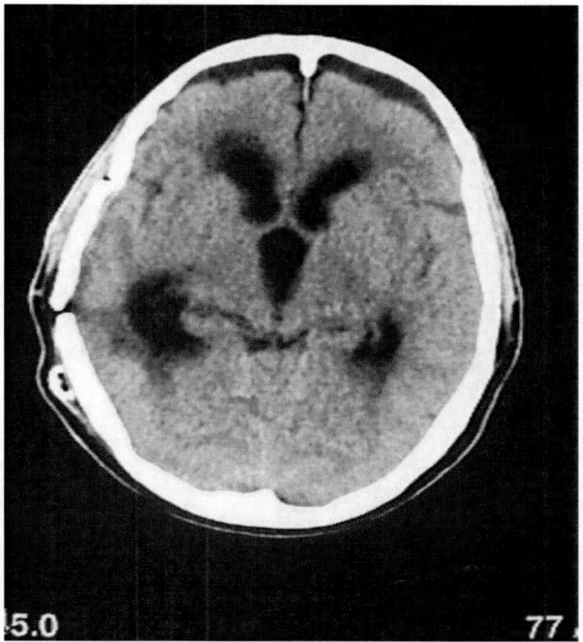

Figure 7. The CT head showing the right temporal craniotomy (done for the removal of a typical EDH following middle meningeal arterial injury) and delayed post traumatic hydrocephalus with periventricular lucencies and frontal subdural collections.

Pediatric brain tumors and maternal brain tumor during pregnancy cause mechanical obstruction of the ventricular system. [13] The tumors blocking the foramen of Monro and anterior third ventricle are sub-ependymal giant cell astrocytoma; gliomas of corpus callosum, anterior third ventricle, thalamic-hypothalamus, optic chiasma or nerve regions; suprasellar craniopharyngioma, arachnoid cysts, etc. The posterior third ventricle and aqueduct may be obstructed by pineal tumors and the vein of Galen aneurysm. The fourth ventricle may be blocked by medulloblastoma, cerebellar astrocytoma, ependymoma and very rarely, by brain stem tumors. In general, these tumors are primarily excised to deal with the ventricular obstruction. Some patients may still develop communicating hydrocephalus and hence need shunting. The routine preoperative shunting in all posterior fossa tumor offers no advantage if the tumor is fully excisable and the obstruction is completely relievable. This is to avoid shunt procedure, tumor dissemination, intratumoral bleeds, and possible upward transtentorial herniation in some of these cases.

However, if there are possibilities of the tumor being partially excised and tumor recurrence /existing tumor dissemination with some persistent obstruction, then the preoperative shunting is undertaken with obvious benefits. In older children, external or internal hydrocephalus needing shunt surgery may be associated with lateral venous sinus occlusion, achondroplasia, craniostenosis (Figure 8), growing skull fracture, osteopetrosis, and posterior fossa cyst (Figure 9). [14]

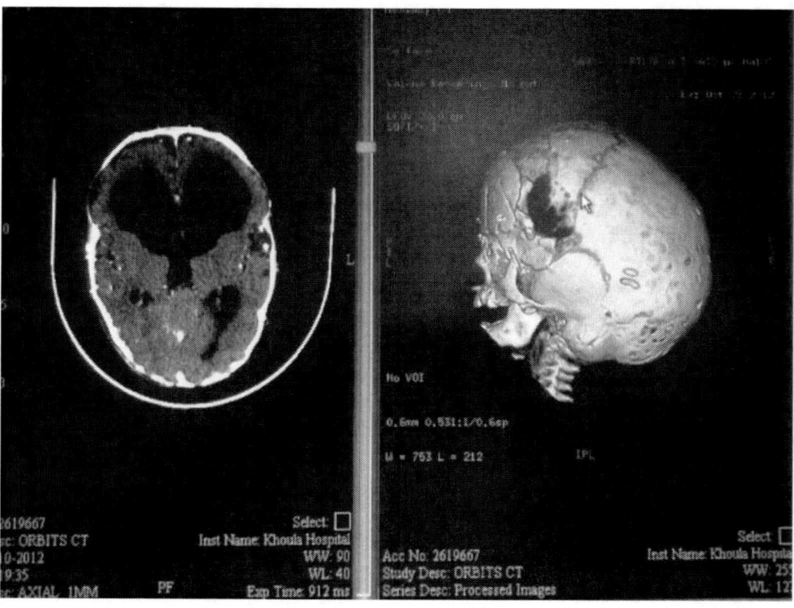

Figure 8. An operated Crouzons syndrome with hydrocephalus which was then treated with VP shunt.

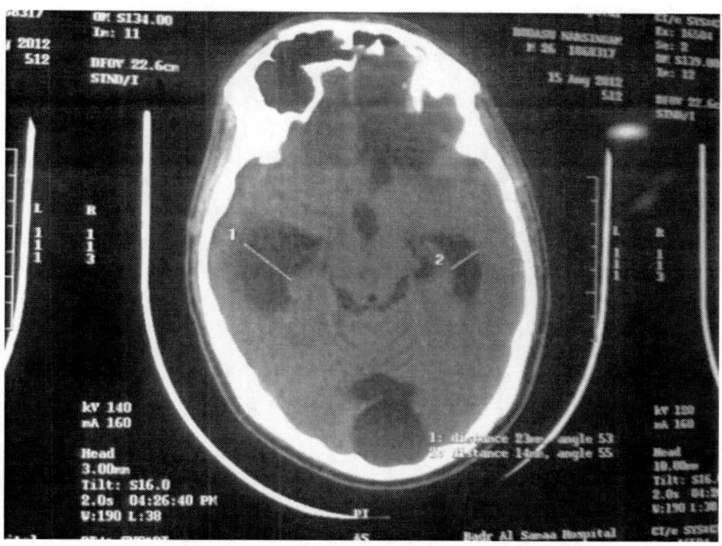

Figure 9. The CT head showing post traumatic hydrocephalus with dilated temporal horns and an incidental posterior fossa arachnoid cyst.

B. Hydrocephalus in adults: [1-7] Nearly in all adult patients, the hydrocephalus is obstructive in nature. The obstruction may be in the ventricles or subarachnoid spaces. The obstruction mainly results in an increased pulsatile CSF pressure in the ventricles overpowering the cerebral compliance and ultimately resulting in a tense dilated or ballooned ventricular system with clinical consequences. "More the intracranial pressure, lesser cerebral blood flow" becomes manifested and needs due surgical attention. The obvious etiological causes of adult hydrocephalus are found in two thirds of cases such as subarachnoid hemorrhage, intra-ventricular hemorrhage, head injury(traumatic IVH and SAH), brain tumors, intracranial infections, aqueduct stenosis and others. In one thirds of cases, the cause may remain undetermined. A significant number of patients with sub arachnoid and intraventricular hemorrhages caused by the cerebral aneurysms, AVMs and hypertension develop hydrocephalus needing neurosurgical management. In the hydrocephalic cases due to intracranial infections, the majority of patient suffers from bacterial meningitis (pyogenic and tubercular) and less commonly, meningeal carcinomatosis and ventriculitis. Rarely, vertebro-basillar insufficiency may cause this. [14]

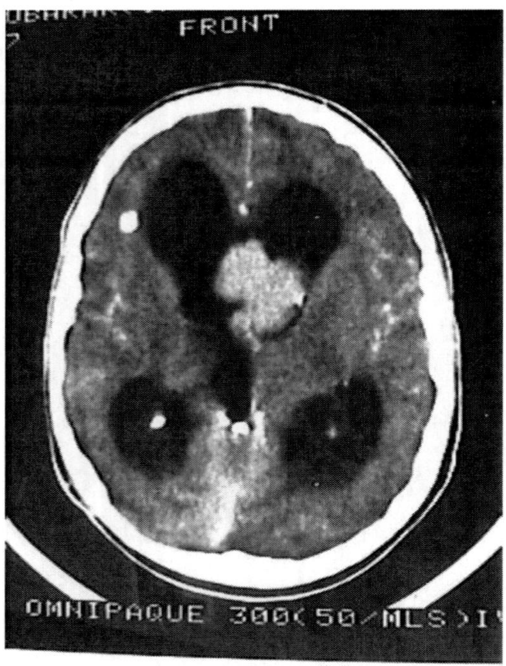

Figure 10. The CT head showing left lateral ventricular –anterior third ventricular glioma causing hydrocephalus in a case of tuberous sclerosis.

The brain tumors (Figures 10 and11), resulting in the obstruction of the CSF circulation, cause hydrocephalus. The commonly occurring tumors are as follows-in the lateral ventricles (sub-ependymal giant cell astrocytomas, choroid plexus papilloma, astrocytoma, ependymomas, meningiomas etc.), third ventricular (colloid cysts, gliomas, choroid plexus papilloma, meningiomas, pineal tumors, parasitic cysts etc); suprasellar region(pituitary adenomas, craniopharyngioma, arachnoid cysts, meningioma, hamartoma, gliomas of the hypothalamus- optic chiasma- optic nerve regions, etc), fourth ventricle (ependymomas, hemangioblastoma, gliomas, choroid plexus papilloma, medulloblastoma, epidermoid and dermoids, parasitic cyst, etc). Brain stem tumors less commonly present with hydrocephalus as compared to other neoplastic lesions. In general, aforementioned obstructive and mass producing tumors are micro-surgically excised. In some cases, the primary excision of these tumors may result in relief in ventricular obstruction; otherwise, the CSF diversion (shunt surgery or endoscopic third ventriculostomy) is performed.

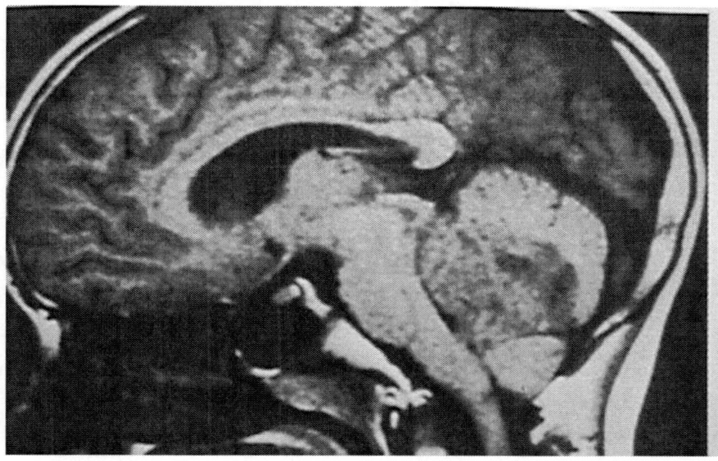

Figure 11. The sagittal T1 weighted MRI scan showing a typical cerebellar medulloblastoma occupying the fourth ventricle.

PATHOPHYSIOLOGY [1-3, 6-8, 9-14]

Patho-physiologically, there is altered CSF dynamics creating a net increase in the hydrostatic pressure on the cerebral parenchyma and thereby resulting in the loss of cerebral parenchymal volume whilst concurrently increasing the volume of the CSF containing spaces in the anatomical cranio-spinal cavities.

1. Pathological processes causing imbalance between CSF production and its absorption with a resultant accumulation of the fluid in the intracranial CSF spaces, primarily in the ventricular system and secondarily in the subarachnoid spaces till both are completely filled with their utmost capacities. If the pathological process is still continuing, the hydrocephalus is termed active/progressive; otherwise termed arrested if the process is inactive. The normal ICP in a neonate may be negative even and in an infant may be as low as 5-7 cm of water and then steadily progressing to 15-18 cm of water in adults. Due to the altered CSF dynamics of production and absorption, there is net accumulation of the fluid in the intracranial CSF spaces resulting in increased intracranial pressure and presenting with the clinical manifestation of the hydrocephalus.

a. Biomechanical profile of the brain in hydrocephalus is well studied by Shapiro et al[15-16] as Pressure –volume index. Volume buffering capacity of the ventricular system is well cited to accommodate a relatively large volume of CSF within with relatively small increases in the ICP till a critical point is reached with the help of visco-elasticity of the brain, opened sutures and fontanellae.

b. Grossly, the rate of production of the CSF is about 1 ml in 3 minutes (20 ml /Hour or 480-500 ml /day). The main production site is choroid plexus (85-90%) in the ventricle where as other sites include ependymal lining of the ventricular system, cerebral capillary endothelium, cells at the root entry zones, and theoretically, from the surfaces of the pial-arachnoid membranes. Initially through the process of ultra-filtration across the non-tight junctions/spaces in the walls of the choroidal capillaries and then via active transport mechanism in the choroid epithelium, the CSF is secreted in all the four ventricular cavities but great majority of the CSF is produced in the lateral ventricles.

c. The CSF is absorbed by the arachnoid villi/granulations projecting in the lateral recesses of the superior sagittal sinus and other venous sinuses. An abnormal high pressure gradient is developed across the site of CSF obstruction: CSF spaces proximal and distal to the obstruction. This results in progressive ventricular dilatation. There is the presence of more than the needed amount of CSF in the cranial cavity with elevated hydrostatic pressure on the brain and vascular tissues with clinical implications. In dynamic events, the CSF may be continually generating and accumulating and in static situations, just occupying the space left by then the current state of the brain tissue. Trans-ependymal absorption is well evident in hydrocephalic states on CT/MRI studies. Rarely, over distension of the ventricular system results rupture at one of its weak spots such as lamina terminalis, supra pineal recess or atrial diverticula bypassing the site of ventricular obstruction and relieving the patient from raised ICP. Unconfirmed speculation of the lymphatic around the cranial nerves and the cerebral vessels is also considered as route of absorption by some investigators.

2. In hydrocephalic cases, raised intracranial pressure and compliance of the brain tissue interact.1-4 If the cerebral compliance (visco-elasticity) overcomes the raised ICP then there is arrested hydrocephalus. Otherwise, Ventricular enlargement results initially in the increase in the cerebral elasticity and later on, gradual increase in the CSF pulse pressure amplitude results in increase in the ventricular size and loss of cerebral mantle. Increase in the ventricular size or ballooning especially of the fourth ventricle may result in the kinking and distortion of the cerebral aqueduct with resultant supra-tentorial tri-ventricular hydrocephalus. Where as in cases of long standing ventriculo- external shunting, the chronically nonfunctioning aqueduct may go into secondary changes with its occlusion. In such cases, trapped fourth ventricle may be seen and this may need surgical intervention. In hydrocephalic babies there may be normal base line intracranial pressure. However, the ICP rises periodically when the baby is asleep especially during slow wave periods and rapid eye movements (REM) phases (Figure 12).

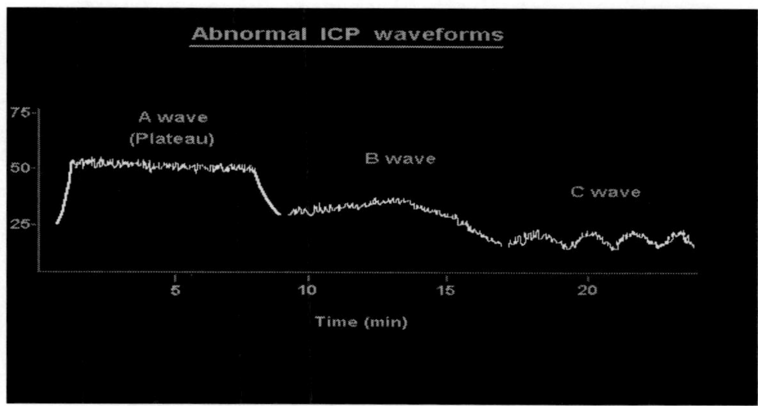

Figure 12. The ICP wave forms are represented in the graphic forms.

3. The type of ventricular dilatation [17 -18] may vary according to the age groups involved. In neonates, premature or young infants, ventricular system in the parieto-occipital region enlarge more preferentially due to more compliant /yielding nature of that part of the brain and overlying cranium as compared to the rigid nature of frontal horns with basal ganglia. In adults the enlargement is far more in the frontal and temporal horns as compared to the body and atria of

the lateral ventricular system. Enlargement of the temporal horns and ballooning of the third ventricle are more sensitive signs of raised intra-ventricular pressure. The stretching of pyramidal fibers especially from the leg area of the brain due to dilated lateral ventricles cause more pronounced ataxia and spasticity as well as their consequent / resultant clinical problems.

4. Parenchymal Histo-Pathological Cahanges: There are many types of pathological changes which vary according to the etiology of the hydrocephalus. For example, the blood and infections in the subarachnoid spaces cause adhesive arachnoiditis and scarring or gluing of arachnoid granulations and their villi (Figure 13). These changes, therefore, result in the loss of passage for the CSF circulation as well as surface for its absorption (absorptive defect) and present with tetra-ventricular communicating hydrocephalus which secondarily cause serious effects on the brain parenchyma. There is gradation of these parenchymal changes as per the degree of the hydrocephalus and raised ICP in relation to their temporal profile.

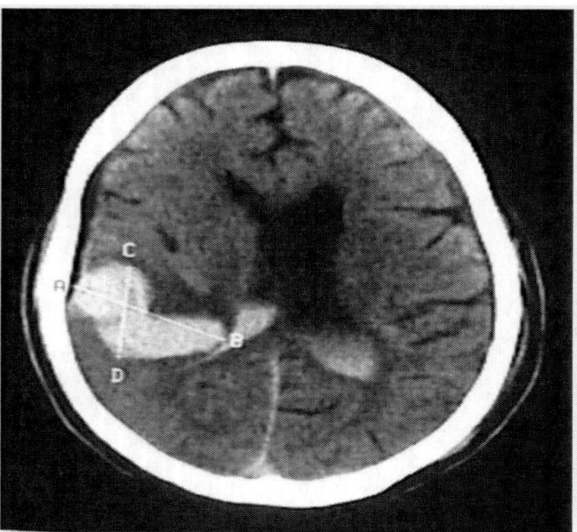

Figure 13. The CT Head showing the IVH bursting into the ventricle and producing mild hydrocephalus.

i. Initially, in acute stages, there is flattening of the ependymal cells with loss of cilia, trans-ependymal seepage of the CSF resulting in the peri-ventricular edema (frontal horn> temporal horn> atria-occipital horn > body of the lateral ventricle) and associated axonal degeneration. Clinically these cases present with progressively increasing ICP.

ii. Later, over a period of time, chronically these changes lead to disruption of the ependymal cellular junctions, astrocytic reactions (astrocytosis) with accommodative interstitial periventricular edema. Clinically these cases present with raised ICP with symptoms suggestive of cognitive impairment.
iii. In advanced stages, there is progressive loss of ependymal lining and its replacement with underlying glial cell processes; loss of branching and spines with evident varicosities in the dendrites as well as interstitial edema with myelin disruption and axonal degenerations ; sub-cortical, peri-ventricular white matter reactive gliosis; neuronal degeneration with loss of cerebral mantle and therefore a picture of cerebral atrophy. Clinically these patients present in advanced state of raised ICP, mantle retardation, developmental delays and spastic limbs.
iv. In terminal stages, the picture of severe loss of cerebral mantle with enlarges ventricles occupying most of the intracranial spaces and distorting and displacing-herniating brain tissues with extremely poor outcome.

5. Biochemical and hormonal changes: Increased concentrations of proteins, fatty acids, hypoxanthine and xanthine, GM1 gangliosides in the CSF due to white matter and neuronal damage as a result of hydrocephalus reported in various studies and their lower or normal concentrations in the cases which were effectively treated. B-transferase and ferritin levels are also measured with no good correlations with the severity. Dilatation of the third ventricle may cause mild to moderate clinically manageable hypothalamic disturbances in form of diabetes insipidus, hyper-natremia, hyper-prolactinemia and reduced growth hormone levels, etc.
6. Psychological and neurological deficits in relation to the hydrocephalus [19-20]

a. Higher mental faculties are affected due to grossly enlarged lateral ventricular system as a whole for a considerable period of time. Interestingly, the grossly dilated frontal and temporal horns cause stretching of the frontal and temporal peri-ventricular fibers and therefore may result in epilepsy, neuro-psychological dysfunctions and altered behavioral patterns. In such cases more, than just one, co-morbid factors (raised ICP, fiber stretching, ischemia, hemorrhage, loss of cerebral mantle) operate to result in cognitive(recognition of the self and surroundings in relation to time, place and person) dysfunctions and conative (psychological attempts of desire, volition and striving) impairment. Non-verbal speech is more affected as compared to its verbal component. In hydrocephalic babies, cortical mantle less than 2.8cm is associated with psychological, social, and physical developmental problems or neuropsychological deficits as compared to the normal cortical mantle of 5cm in healthy babies. [20]

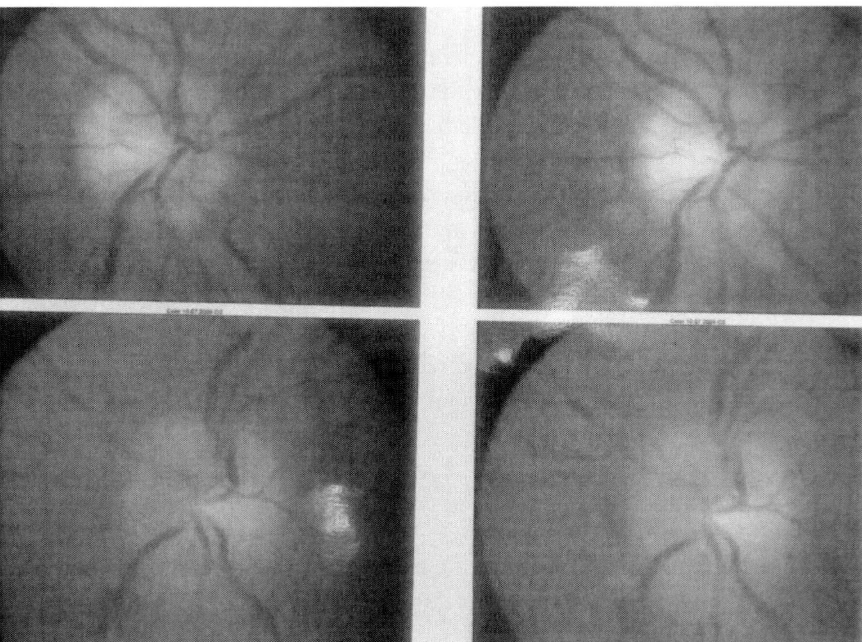

Figure 14. (a, b, c, and d; left to right): Fundoscopy showing severe progressive papilledema.

b. Cranial nerve dysfunctions: [1-8] Although, the severely dilated lateral ventricles may flattened the olfactory bulbs and tracts, smell sensations are largely spared in hydrocephalus. Papilledema (Figures 14-16) is a well recognized clinical sign of raised ICP due to any cause except that the causative pathology should not be directly compressing that optic nerve (obliterating the subarachnoid spaces around the optic nerve and compressing the optic fibers and thus primarily resulting in compressive optic atrophy). Delayed visual impairment or progressive loss of vision is well recognized in cases of advanced papilledema due to compression, edema, ischemia etc. Anisocoria (unequal pupils) / Hutchinson's pupil (one dilated pupil) or bilateral dilated pupils are well known in cases of transtentorial herniation of the uncus of the temporal lobe or trans-foraminal tonsillar -medullary herniation due to highly significant ventricular dilatation under increased intra-ventricular CSF pressure and the resultant brain shifts.

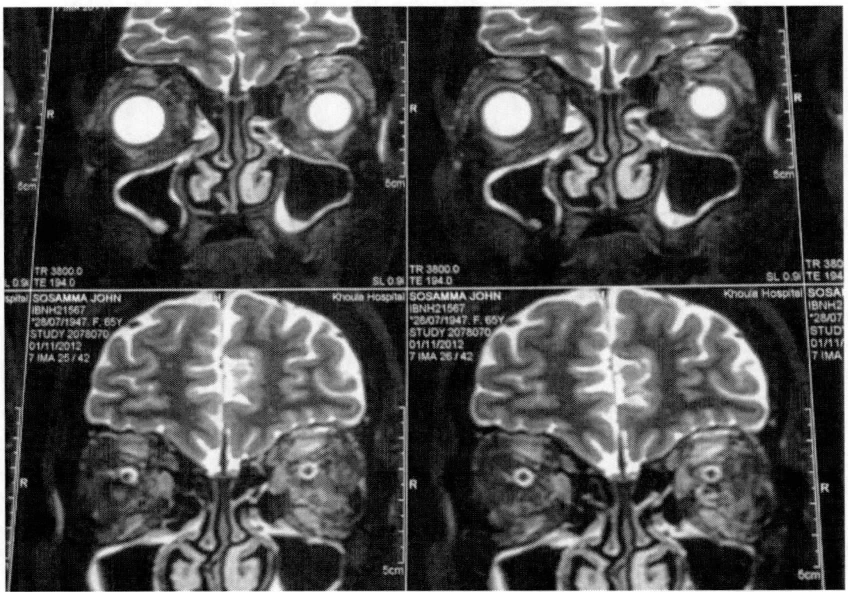

Figure 15. (a,b,c, and d): The coronal T2 weighted MRI scan showing the well formed dilated perioptic subarachnoid spaces.

Minor abnormalities of papillary inequalities are more commonly noted as with brain tumors (Figures 17-18). Sun setting(or sun rising) eye sign is mainly due to the dilated lateral ventricular pressure effects on the thin orbital roof plates as well as the direct pressure effects of the dilated ballooned third ventricle on the tectum of the midbrain and peri-aqueductal gray matter. Typical picture is that of downward displacement of the eyeballs, upward retraction of the upper eyelids, paralyzed upward gaze (Perinaud's syndrome), divergence of the eyeballs with impaired convergence, etc. Sixth, third and fourth cranial nerve palsies in decreasing order are well known in cases of significant hydrocephalus.

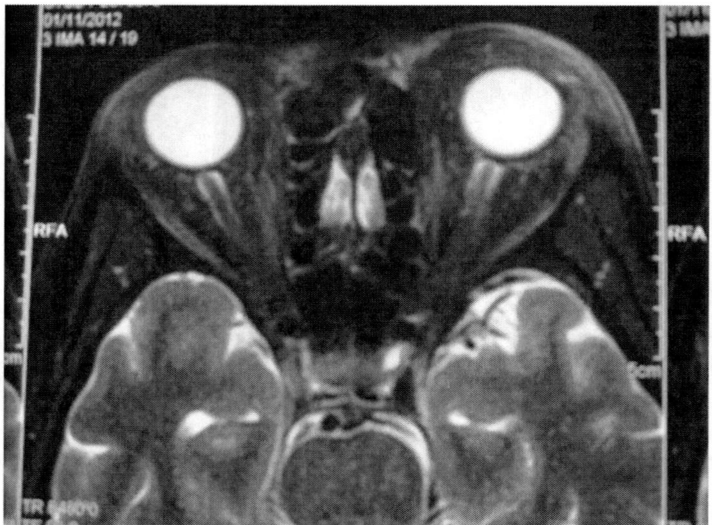

Figure 16. The T2 weighted MRI scan of the orbits showing well formed subarachnoid spaces around the optic nerves.

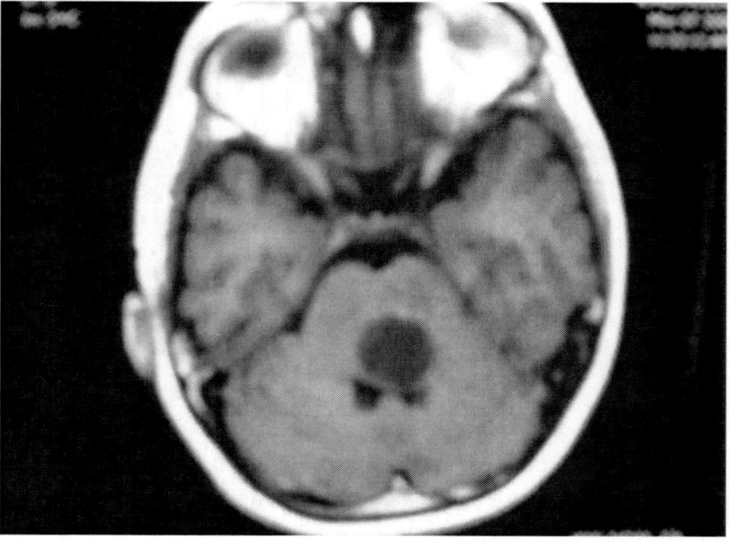

Figure 17. The T1 weighted image of the MRI scan showing a low attenuation lesion in the brain stem. The brain stem gliomas rarely cause hydrocephalus.

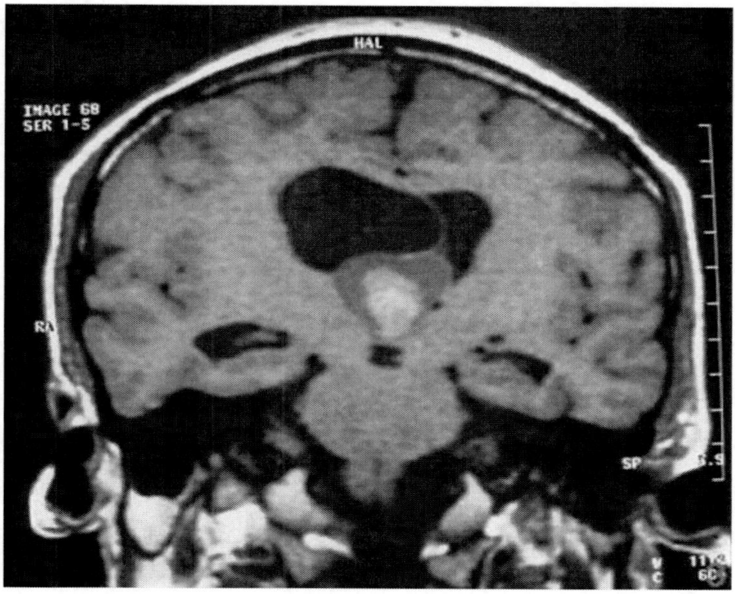

Figure 18. The coronal MRI scan showing asymmetric lateral ventricular dilatation due to a third ventricular tumor.

Supranuclear facial paresis, vestibule- cochlear symptoms (tinnitus, imbalance, hearing impairment) and the disturbances of the lower cranial nerves and trigeminal system are occasionally noted.

c. Sensory motor abnormalities affecting the body and the limbs: Sensory findings are more difficult to be evaluated than the motor ones in the early developmental periods: neonates and infants. Grossly the pain sensations are rarely affected due to ventricular dilation. However, if the hydromyelia is associated with it then this may result in suspended loss of pain sensations with variable loss of touch and other sensations better evaluated in adults. The more pronounced effects are there on the motor system of the body and the limbs. Hydrocephalic fits where the baby appears awake conscious with severe decorticate or decerebrate rigidity with grossly dilated ventricles with impending herniations and these conditions are needing immediate attention. Ophisthotonus position is not rare in such severe cases. The more common presentations are spastic paraparesis with variable scissoring in infants; whereas, in adults only spasticity without paraparesis may be noted.

Dilated lateral and third ventricles(affecting the white matter pyramidal fibers as well highly stretched anterior cerebral arteries with corpus callosum over the ballooned third ventricle), hydromyelia, myelo-dysplasia with Arnold Chiari malformations are some commonly implicated co-morbid factors for the motor dysfunctions. Many of these motor sensory symptoms and signs may resolve with the appropriate management of hydrocephalus and its associated conditions such as hydromyelia, Arnold Chiari malformation and myelodysplasia.

CLINICAL PRESENTATIONS [3, 6-7,17-20]

Hydrocephalus is diagnosed currently with great ease using modern clinico-radiological studies such as ultrasound studies, Computed tomography and MRI studies. However, purely for the clinical purposes, there are variations in the clinical presentations of these cases according to their age groups which need to be aware of and recognized early enough for an effective management.

1. Fetal hydrocephalus: Intrauterine diagnosis of the hydrocephalus due to developmental anomalies or intrauterine infection/trauma is made using ultrasound studies during periodic preterm obstetric follow up visits.
2. Neonatal /infantile hydrocephalus: Prematurity with intracranial hemorrhage, Myelodysplasia with Arnold-Chiari malformation, peri-natal CNS infections, congenital malformations, etc.

Initially, there is a progressive enlargement of the head (macrocephaly) due to gradually increasing ventriculomegaly with cranial suture separation / diastases with no features of raised ICP in neonates and infants. This is very well assessed on the head circumference chart against the age groups in male and female infants. Acute hydrocephalus will present with irritable baby with excessive high pitched crying, non-acceptance of feeds with projectile vomits, bulging fontanels with some separation of sutures and dilated scalp veins (Figure 19) as well as sun setting eye sign.

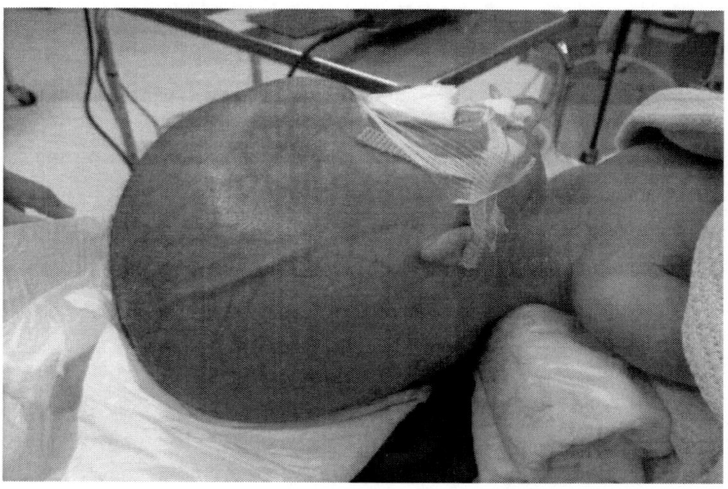

Figure 19. A case with severe hydrocephalus showing stretched scalp and prominently engorged scalp veins.

Later on, if the clinical progress is more gradual then in addition to the aforementioned features, there are features of raised intracranial pressure such as subdued responses, drowsiness, non-acceptance of the feeds, projectile vomiting, irritability, lethargy, lack of active responses and bulging fontanels prominent scalp veins and sun setting sign of the eyes with upward gaze paresis in infants.

3. In the older children, the symptomatology may include headaches, altered mental status, confusion, decreased responsiveness, irritability-agitation, imbalance, incontinence, spastic limbs with and without scissoring, etc.
4. In adults: There is a well recognized tetrad of clinical features of raised ICP: headaches, vomiting, episodic visual obscurations and papilledema with retinal venous engorgement and loss of venous pulsations. Morning headaches and the projectile vomits suggest raised ICP due to reduced CSF drainage in the supine, recumbent position during the sleep at night. Ataxia, visual disturbances (impairment of visual acuity, reduction in visual fields, diplopia, abducens palsy, Perinaud's syndrome, etc), disorientation, impairment of recent memory or disturbance of higher mental function, and focal neurological deficits in the limbs are carefully assessed and investigated. The patients with SAH, IVH, meningitis, brain tumors,

and traumatic brain injury should have an expectant OPD follow up to detect delayed occurrence of the hydrocephalus if it is not present in their acute states.

5. In elderly patients, [5] the presentation may be more interesting with no features of raised ICP but with the features of so-called clinical triad of symptoms (DAI) of normal pressure hydrocephalus: dementia (confusion, lack of insight, inability to analyze and appropriately respond with and without emotional lability), ataxia (imbalance whilst walking and using hands) and incontinence (Figure 20).

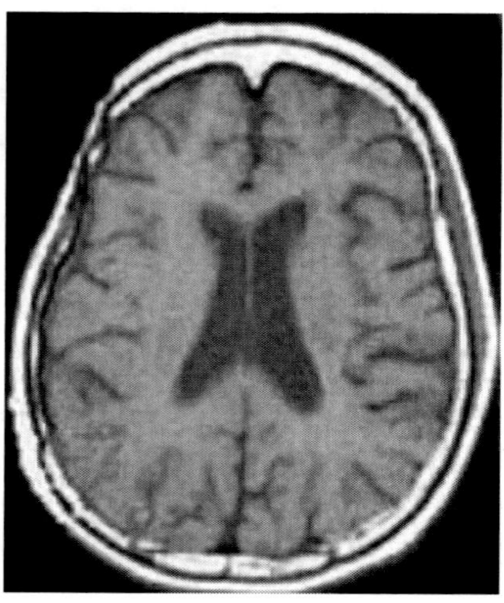

Figure 20. The T1 weighted axial MRI scan showing mildly dilated ventricle with opened cerebral sulci in a typical case of normal pressure hydrocephalus.

Clinical Diagnosis and Investigations [1-3,7,21-22]

In initial neonatal period, first, the head size usually decreases with concurrent transient increase in the ventricular size due to the loss of normal salt and water from the body as well as with some decrease in ICP. Then the head size increases due to the period of concurrent brain growth with some reduction in the ventricular size and normalization of the ICP. Following this period, then there is correlative relationship between the head size and brain growth during the developmental period and nearly a steady state thereafter.

It is far easier in the neonates and infants to diagnose hydrocephalus on the clinical grounds than in the adults and elderly as the presenting features of raised ICP may be same or may mimic each other in plethora of etiologies.

A. In neonates, a large head or progressively enlarging head will always point towards suspicion of hydrocephalus; but interestingly, in small number of hydrocephalic babies, even the features of normal head circumference with slack anterior fontanel but gross ventricular dilatation are not unusual. Ultrasound studies of the head using sonographic criteria of the measurement of various parts of the ventricular system are of paramount importance in its diagnosis.
B. Infantile hydrocephalus is suspected clinically in any infant with rapid increase in its head circumference as per the plotting of head circumference curves on the standardized head circumference measurement (curves) charts as per the age and the sex. With some differences in the male and female babies; grossly, the normal size is about 33-35 cm at birth and then there is an increase of about 0.7 to 1.0 cm /month for the first six months of life and thereafter 0.5 cm /month for next six month period. In the second year there is an increase in size of about 0.25cm/month to reach a head size of about 45 cm at the end of 24 months.

Neuro-Radiological Studies [2-9]

This has revolutionized the management of the CNS pathologies with least possible morbidities and mortality. Some techniques have become as a matter of routine investigations such as ultra-sonographic studies, high resolution spiral computed tomography (CT Scans) with MIP reconstructions, digital substraction angiography (DSA) and Magnetic Resonance imaging (MRI Scans). Whereas some other techniques, which were routine in the past, are not favored anymore due to their obvious disadvantages i.e., such as pneumo-encephalography (PEG), oil based or water soluble contrast enhanced ventriculo-cisternography, radionuclide cisternography, invasive myelography, etc.

A. Ultrasonography (Figure 21) remains highly useful and successful screening investigation for the hydrocephalus in cases with open anterior fontanel. It is a non-invasive, non-sedating, OPD based, bedside, user and consumer friendly, least time consuming, real time, economical with reproducible findings with no obvious related morbidities and mortality. It shows clearly the state of the cerebral mantle, ventricles and some idea about the intracranial pathology. To elucidate the cause further, the other neuro-imaging studies may be undertaken.

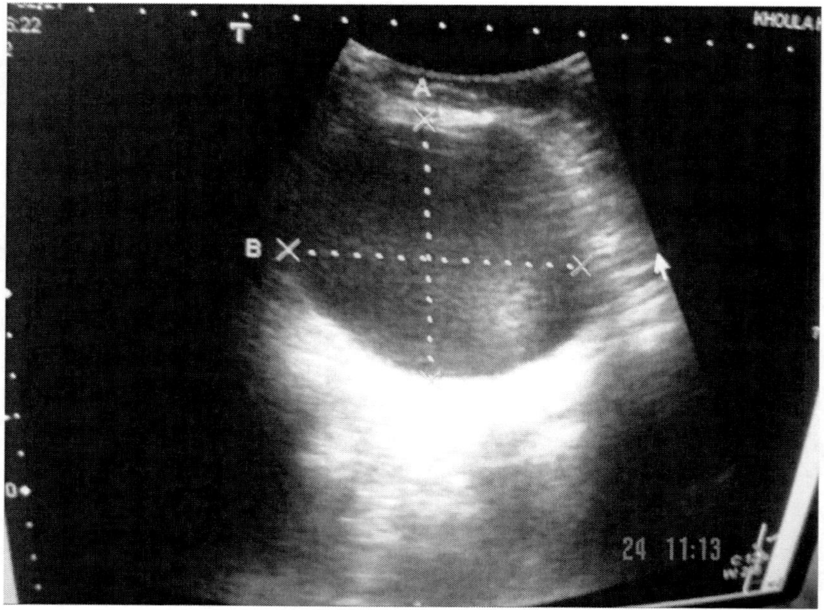

Figure 21. Ultrasonography showing a large CSF filled cyst cavity.

The CT scan and MRI scans are highly useful, successful and informative techniques with some limitations and morbidities especially X-ray related concerns with the CT scans and GA related concerns in MRI scans so as to avoid artifacts. Periodic studies show that there is a progressive enlargement of the ventricular system with rounding of the ventricular crevices such as frontal / occipital /temporal horns and trans-ependymal seepage of the CSF, thinning of the cortical-subcortical mantle, stretching of the cerebral vasculature/ependymal lining/corpus callosum and concurrently there is progressive compromise/ obliteration of the subarachnoid spaces and CSF cisterns.

The term 'Hydrocephalus ex vacuo' is used if the ventricular system and subarachnoid spaces are enlarged due to the cerebral atrophy seen on the neuro-imaging studies. Whereas, if the brain is normal and subarachnoid spaces are compromised with enlargement of the ventricles and stretching of the neuro-vascular tissues including the ependymal linings, then the hydrocephalus is defined radiologically as an active hydrocephalus with significantly raised intracranial pressure.

The CT head scan (Figures 22-24), with and without contrast, is most commonly used in emergency situation to assess the ventricular size and identifying the causative pathology. Further characterization of the offending brain lesion is done with the help of the MRI scan, MR Angiography and MR spectroscopy. The CSF flow can also be measured across the aqueduct with MR flow void technique.

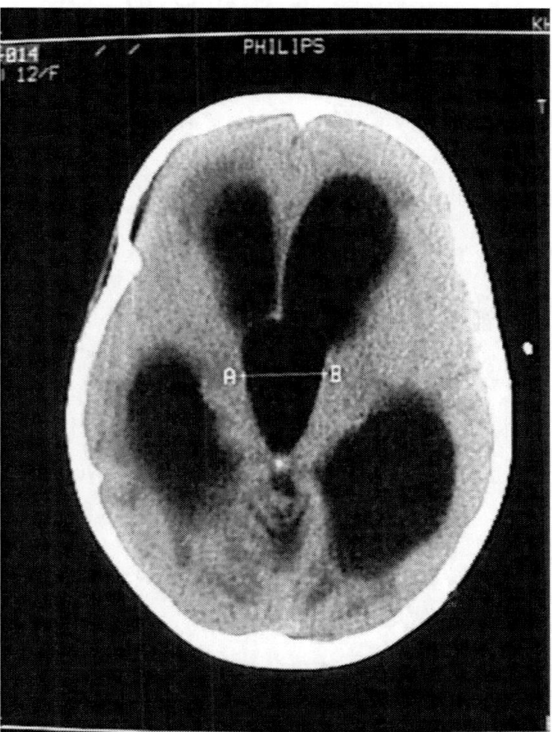

Figure 22. The CT head showing massive (obstructive) hydrocephalus with ballooned third ventricle (ideal for endoscopic third ventriculostomy).

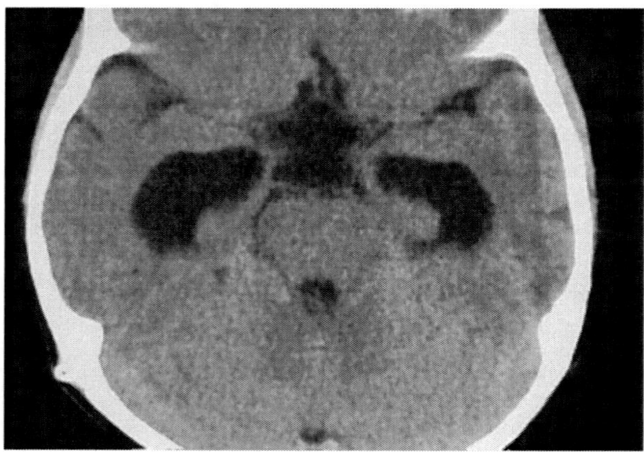

Figure 23. The CT head large dilated temporal horns suggestive of massive hydrocephalus.

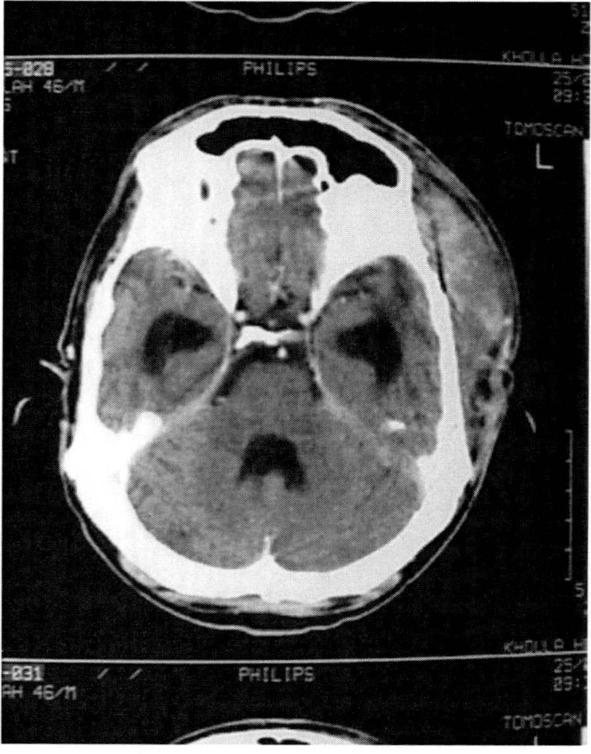

Figure 24. The CT Head showing dilated temporal horns of the lateral ventricles with normal fourth ventricle and supra-sellar cistern.

MANAGEMENT OF HYDROCEPHALUS [1-6, 9-12, 21-23]

Hydrocephalus (CSF under increased ICP) is causing progressive adverse effects on the brain. Hence delay in its management may result in significant functional deterioration. Timely management of the symptomatic hydrocephalus is, therefore, highly rewarding.

The management of hydrocephalus surrounds following three interlinked principles

1. To halt the progressive enlargement of the ventricular size
2. To normalize the raised ICP
3. To halt progressive neurological deterioration and pave the way for clinical recovery

In an established case of hydrocephalus, the primary concern is continued CSF production and correspondingly increasing ICP.

1. Medical Considerations [1-7, 22-24]

The CSF production is an active energy consuming process. Therefore, it can be altered with the help of the medicinal or pharmacological management to some extent. The medications which can reduce CSF production are as follows-acetazolamide (carbonic anhydrase inhibitor), furosemide (affecting chloride cellular mechanism), cardiac glycosides (Na-K-ATPase pump inhibition), isosorbide, topiramate, etc. Infants were given acetazolamide 100 mg/kg/day and furosemide 1mg/kg/day with good results in about 50% cases with mild hydrocephalus.

In cases of prematurity with intracerebral hematoma and intraventricular rupture/hemorrhage, serial lumbar puncture may yield good results. Combination of acetazolamide and serial lumbar punctures had been successfully tried in some cases of post bacterial meningitic hydrocephalus. External compression of the head has been abandoned due to lack of any clinical benefits.

There are no known pharmacological drugs which can increase the process of CSF circulation in the CSF spaces and absorption at the arachnoid villi and granulations.

2. Surgical Considerations [17-21, 24-26]

There is plethora of surgical options in the management of the active hydrocephalus but none is successful in all cases. The basis of surgical intervention is either effective reduction in the CSF production or the effective CSF diversion to a safe site with least possible morbidity and mortality.

A. Surgical excision or fulguration of the choroid plexus of the lateral ventricles: Pathological conditions such as hypertrophic choroid plexus or choroid plexus papilloma give rise to significantly increased production of the CSF and can be treated with surgical excision or coagulation to reduce CSF production. However, it is largely given up in the era of CSF shunting.
B. Direct microscopic / percutaneous / endoscopic third ventriculostomy via the floor of the third ventricle or lamina terminalis in the management of non-communicating, obstructive hydrocephalus, i.e. hydrocephalus associated with brain tumors.
C. CSF Shunting is the most commonly used and is reliable means of managing hydrocephalus. Nearly, all patients with communicating hydrocephalus (absorptive defects) are treated with extracranial shunting procedures.

1. Intracranial CSF diversion procedures

   a. Torkildsen procedure: shunting the lateral ventricles to cisterna magna-upper cervical subarachnoid spaces in patient with third ventricular or aqueductal obstruction.
   b. Open/percutaneous canalization of the aqueduct-a technique with high morbidity, not advisable if alternative safer treatment methods are available,
   c. Lateral ventriculo-venous sinus shunt-mostly unreliable

2. Extracranial CSF diversion procedures: following methods are more reliable –

   A. Ventriculo-peritoneal shunts-most reliable and dependable
   B. Shunting outside the peritoneum when VP shunting not feasible

i. Lumbo-peritoneal shunt
ii. Ventriculo-atrial shunt
iii. ventriculo-pleural shunt

SOME OF THE AFOREMENTIONED PROCEDURES WHICH ARE CURRENTLY DONE ARE AS FOLLOWS [1-3]

1. Endoscopic Third Ventriculostomy [1-9,16, 25-29]

Earlier, Victor Darwin [27] and then in 1922, Walter Dandy described third ventriculostomy (a CSF communication between the third ventricle and the inter-peduncular cistern via a surgically created hole in the floor of the third ventricle) [28] for the management of hydrocephalus associated with the aqueduct stenosis.

In 1923, Mixter did third ventriculostomy using ventriculoscope which he had passed from the anterior fontanel to the foramen of Monro then to the floor of the third ventricle. [29] A flexible sound was then used to perforate the third ventricular floor to enter into the inter-peduncular cistern. In 1939, Stookey and scarff had used a sub-frontal approach to make an opening in the lamina terminalis. [30-32] Milhorat et al revealed in autopsy studies that CSF spaces are potentially open but mechanically compressed in cases of congenital hydrocephalus. Kelly et al described CT stereotactic third ventriculostomy. [30]

Currently, the advances in neuro-endoscopy have made third ventriculostomy (NTV) a safer routine procedure (Figures-25-30) in many cases of obstructive hydrocephalus with decreased mortality and morbidity. The main Indications for NTV are symptomatic obstructive hydrocephalus in cases of aqueduct stenosis, brain stem lesions, Dandy-Walker syndrome, Arnold- Chiari malformation, myelo-dysplasia, pineal tumors, fourth ventricular tumors, supra-sellar arachnoid cyst, etc.

To perform NTV [27-32] on these cases,a sagittal MR images showing ballooning of third ventricle is usually needed along with the details of the lesion per say. During the procedure, one can use either a flexible or a rigid endoscope with working ports.

Via a small frontal burr hole, the neuro-endoscope is introduced in the lateral ventricle and then in the foramen of Monro. On reaching the floor of the third ventricle, a small ventriculostomy is performed in an area bounded by mammilary bodies on the postero-lateral sided and pituitary infundibulam and tuber cinereum anteriorly.

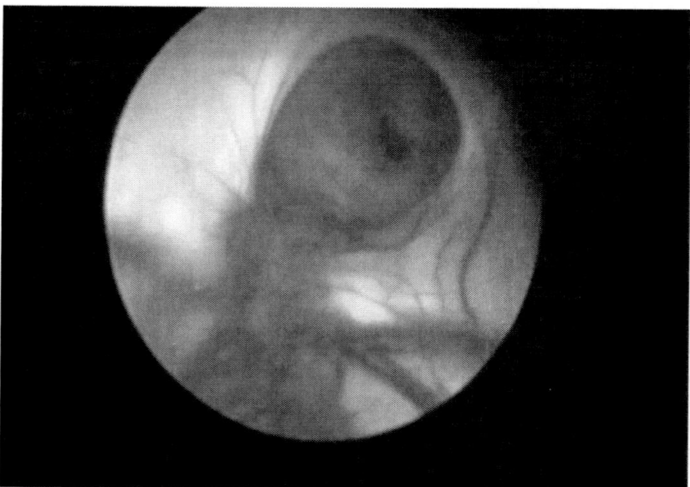

Figure 25. The endoscopic view of the foramen of Monro showing choroid plexus with thalamostiate and septal veins entering into the roof of the third ventricle as well as the middle part of the floor of the third ventricle is also visualized.

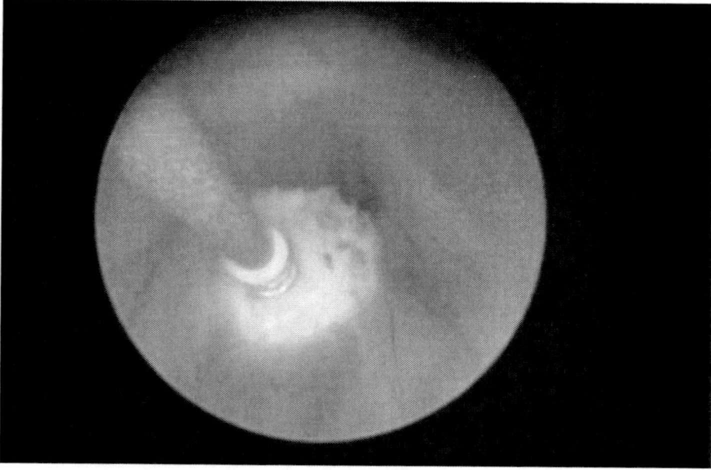

Figure 26. The endoscopic view of the third ventriculostomy which is being dilated with a fogarty balloon catheter.

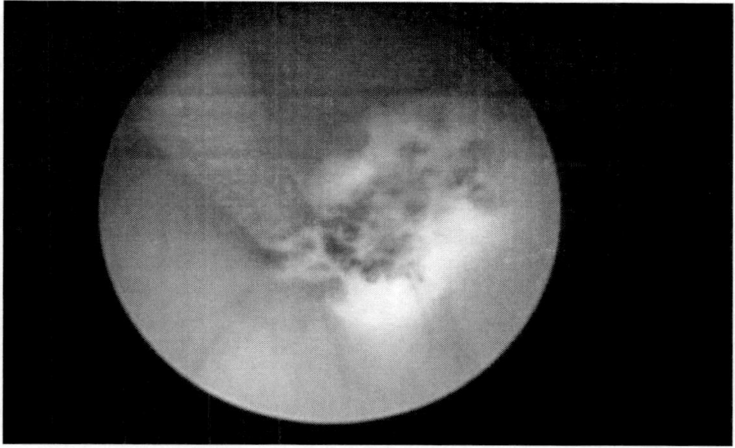

Figure 27. The endoscopic view showing the fogarty balloon catheter in the supasellar cistern for further dilatation and opening of the passages.

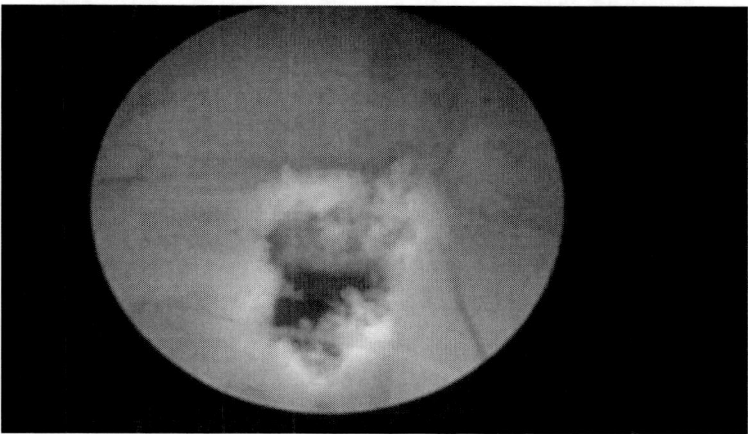

Figure 28. The endoscopic view showing a well formed third ventriculostomy.

The osteum is then enlarged with the balloon catheter. The CSF is seen flowing freely through the ventriculostomy at surgery. The procedure is also used for reconstruction of the ostomy if it gets blocked over a period of time. However, if third ventriculostomy is not successful; then the appropriate shunt surgery is performed in such cases.

Endoscopic or direct extirpation of choroid plexus also is a suggested treatment of the hydrocephalus. There is a growing literature on neuro-endoscopy treatment. [33-37]

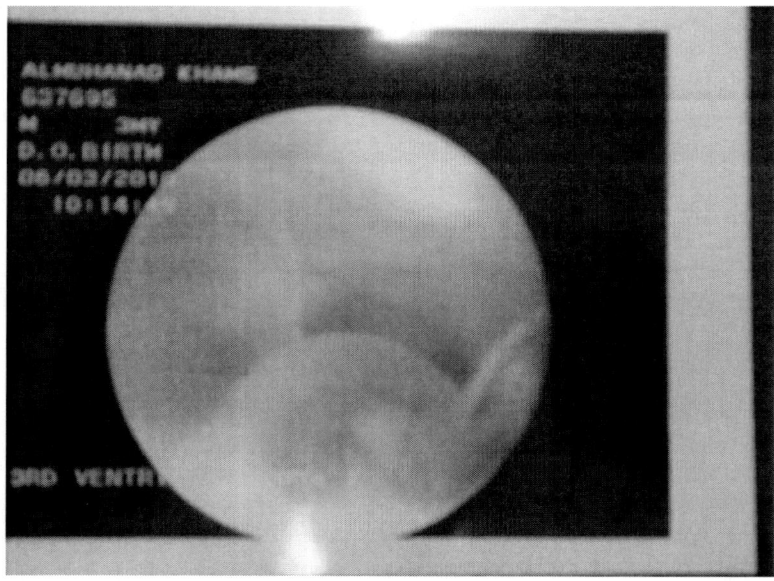

Figure 29. Endoscopic views of the basilar system and both oculomotor nerves in the inter-peduncular cistern.

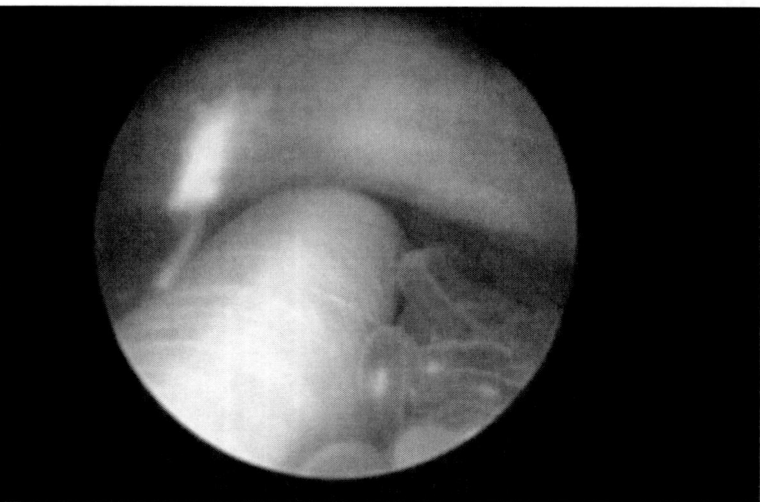

Figure 30. The endoscopic view showing the structures in the pre-pontine cistern: dorsum sellae and clival area, basilar artery and brain stem perforators.

2. Fetal Shunt Surgery

Intrauterine placement of the shunt has been tried in anecdotal cases with variable experiences. Such surgery faces many problems related to false ultrasound diagnosis, unreliability of progressive nature of the hydrocephalus; technical challenges during surgery, unreliable functioning of the shunt system, post infective hydrocephalus, fetal viability concerns (fetal amniotic lecithin-to- sphingomyelin ratio) due to severe associated malformations, etc. In some instances, hydrocephalic viable baby is delivered by cesarean section and then it is subjected to the formal shunt surgery.

3. Shunt Surgery: In Pediatirc and Adult Patients [1-4,7-12, 18-23,38]

Post natal shunting has also been tried in all other possible combinations: from the cerebral ventricle to the spaces in the head (scalp, mastoids), face (Stevens duct), thorax (pleura, thoracic duct), abdomen (peritoneal cavity, colon, intestine, ureters, Gall bladder etc), pelvis (fallopian tube, urinary bladder), etc but without much success apart from the following four extracranial CSF diversion procedures (Figures 31-33): the VP shunt, VA shunt, V-PL shunt and LP shunt.

A standard shunt system has a ventricular or proximal catheter with multiple holes for about 2 cm near the tip for the CSF to come into it, a connecting chamber for pumping (or aspirating/injecting, assessing patency and pressure measurements), a valve allowing unidirectional flow of the CSF, and a distal catheter for the extra- cranial space where it is intended to drain CSF for its absorption. Many varieties of the shunt systems are made available for use according to the patients need, as well as institutes /operators preferences. [39]

I. Ventriculo-Peritoneal (VP) Shunts [1-14,40]

This procedure is routine, first choice, all over the neurosurgical centers due to its ease of placement and functional reliability as compared to the other alternatives (Figures 34-36).

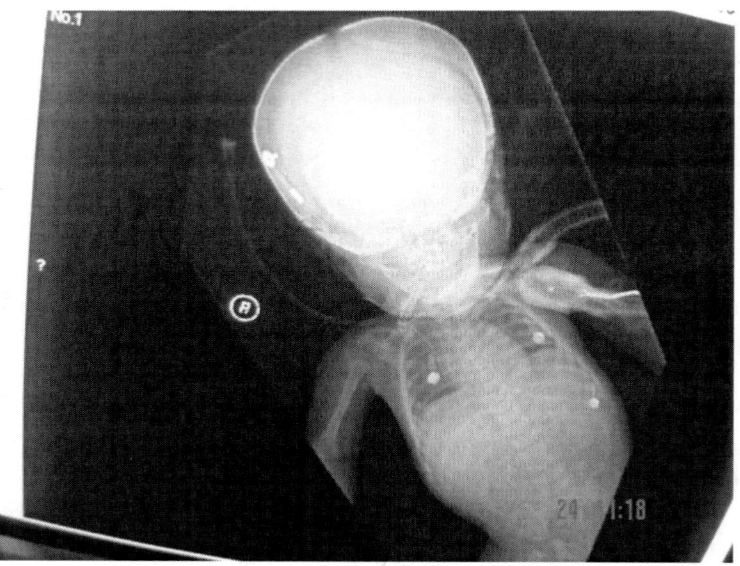

Figure 31. The plain X-rays showing the disconnection of the proximal end which is floating in the right lateral ventricle.

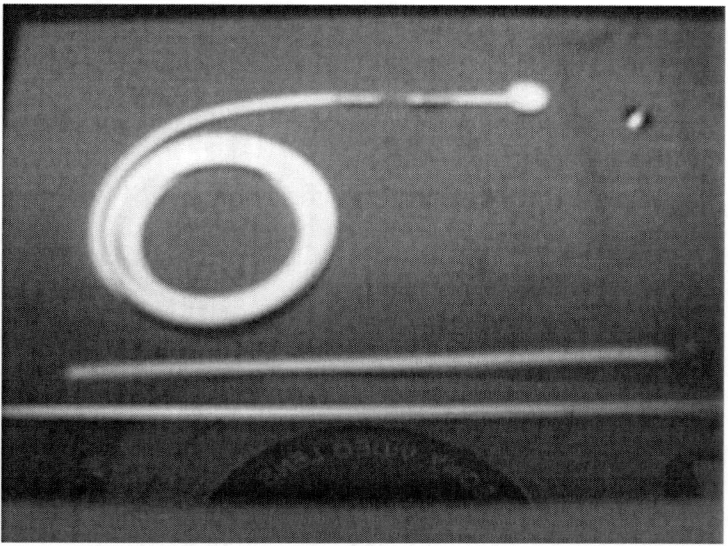

Figure 32. The components of a typical shunt system: The chamber attached to the valve and the distal catheter above and distal catheter in the middle as well as subcutaneous tunneller at the bottom.

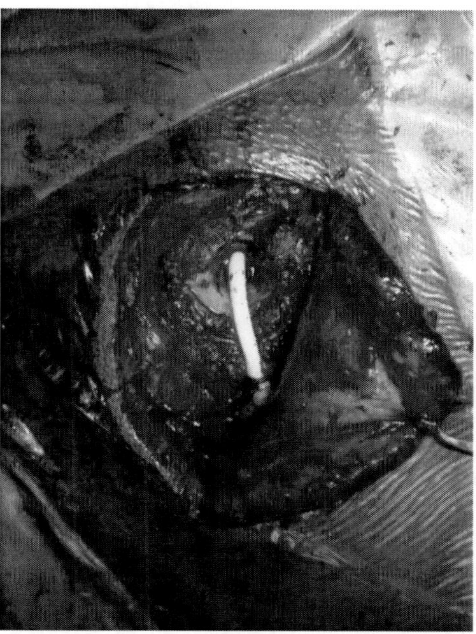

Figure 33. The per-operative picture showing the burr hole and proximal catheter placed in the ventricle.

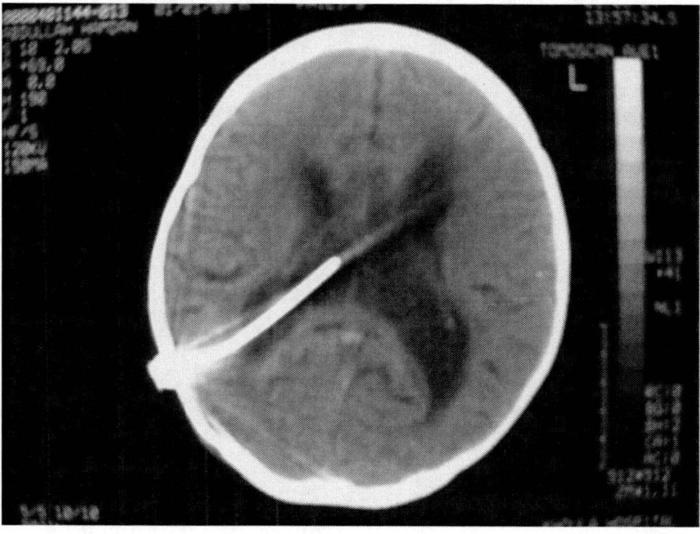

Figure 34. The CT head showing a well functioning proximal end with reduction in the size of the lateral ventricles and appearance of the cerebral cortical sulci.

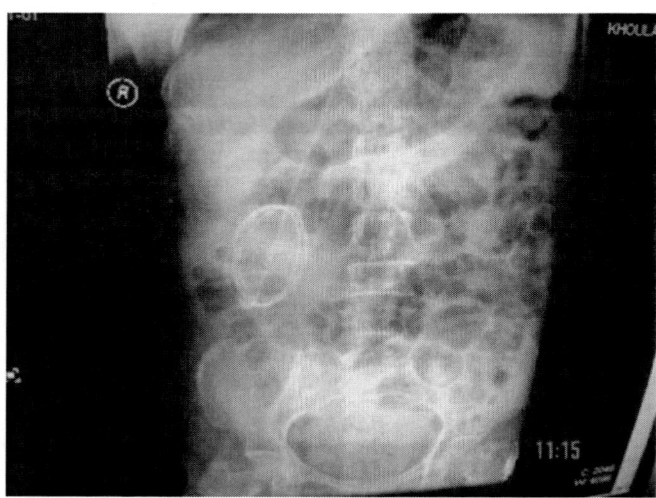

Figure 35. The plain X-rays of the abdomen showing the peritoneal catheter in the immediate post operative period with gaseous abdominal distension.

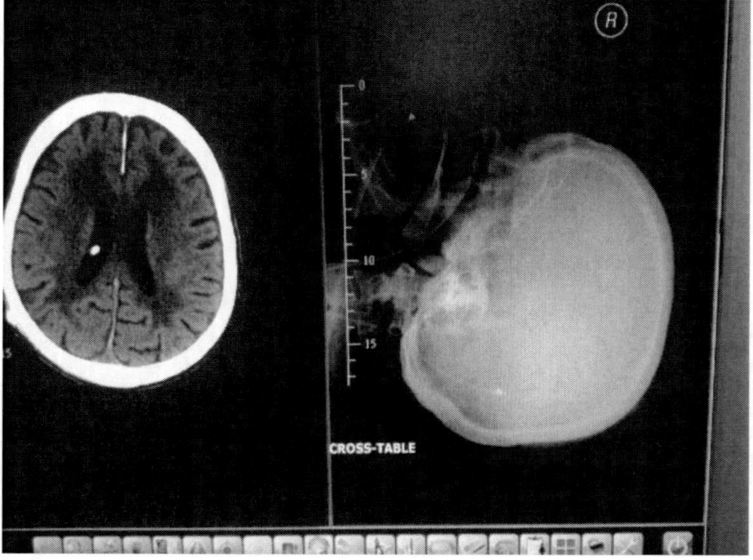

Figure 36. A case of NPH treated with programmable shunt system.

Ventricular catheter is introduced through a parietal/frontal burr hole into the lateral ventricle preferably into the frontal horn to avoid blockage of the catheter holes with the choroid plexus. The chamber in placed either on the burr hole or a little away from it and then connected to the unidirectional valve. The distal peritoneal catheter is placed subcutaneously connected to the valve and its distal part with the tip (40-50 cm to accommodate for the future growth period) into the abdominal cavity through a sub-costal or a midline incision. In a great majority of cases, this procedure is satisfactory.

II. Lumbo-Peritoneal (LP) Shunt: [41]

This [also called as theco-peritoneal (TP)shunt] is a second choice in the management of the communicating hydrocephalus mainly in adults (Figures 37-38) in following situations: when the ventricular size is small and the ICP is high, presence of burr hole site infection, anterior chest wall infection or when the other methods are not readily available in adults. Percutaneous technique is used for the insertion of the lumbar catheter in the lumbar cistern (usually between L3 to 5 level) and then the placement of the valve with catheter subcutaneously in the loin area and the distal end in the abdominal cavity by open/percutaneous technique.It is also very useful in some cases of benign intracranial hypertension, Slit ventricles, cranial CSF leaks and syringomyelia.

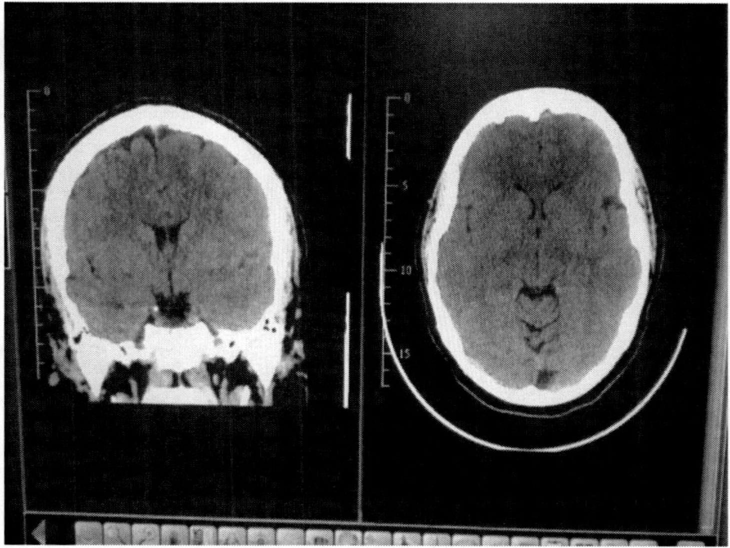

Figure 37. The CT scan films showing the typical features of the slit ventricles and mimics benign intracranial hypertension.

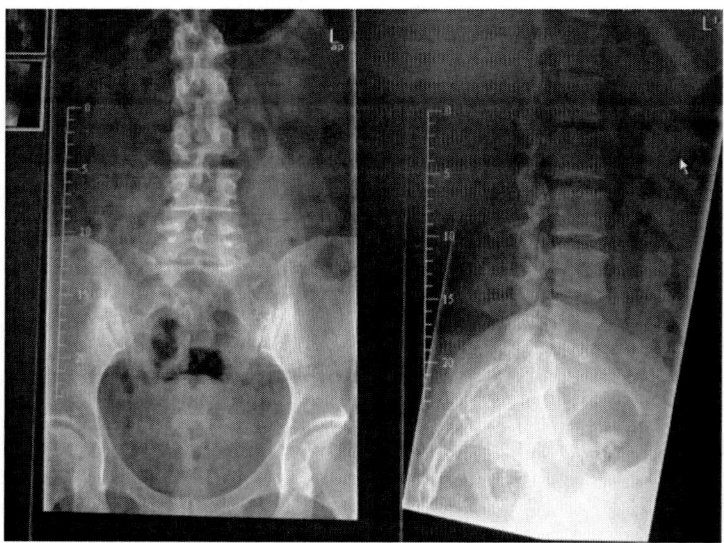

Figure 38. The AP and Lateral X-rays views of the lumbar spine showing the LP shunt in place.

III. Ventriculo-Atrial (Va) Shunts [1-12, 19,22-24]

This is one of the best choices in neonates, infants and children, when the abdominal cavity is not available for shunting due to whatever cause (Figure 39). The insertion of the ventricular catheter is performed same as in VP shunt through a parietal/frontal burr hole into the lateral ventricle. Then, the shunt chamber is placed either on the burr hole or a little away from it and then connected to the unidirectional valve. The distal atrial catheter is placed subcutaneously connected to the valve and its distal part with the tip {at the 7thor 8th intercostals space or ninth thoracic (T9) vertebral body as seen on per-operative AP Chest X-ray with water soluble contrast injection into the catheter} into the right atrium of the heart (through a cervical incision via a common facial vein or an internal jugular vein).

Central venous pressure recording are noted during the insertion of the catheter which may confirm the position of the catheter tip and the pressure recording helps in avoiding ventricular placement of the catheter tip. In a majority of cases, this procedure is also satisfactory. Apart from the chest X-rays and CVP monitoring during the surgery, the ECG and ultrasonography may be helpful. Whereas post operatively X-ray chest and echocardiography may help in confirming the positions of the catheter tip in the right atrium. Rarely the patient may need multiple revisions and even the need for direct implantation of the catheter into the right atrium when no other solution is feasible etc.

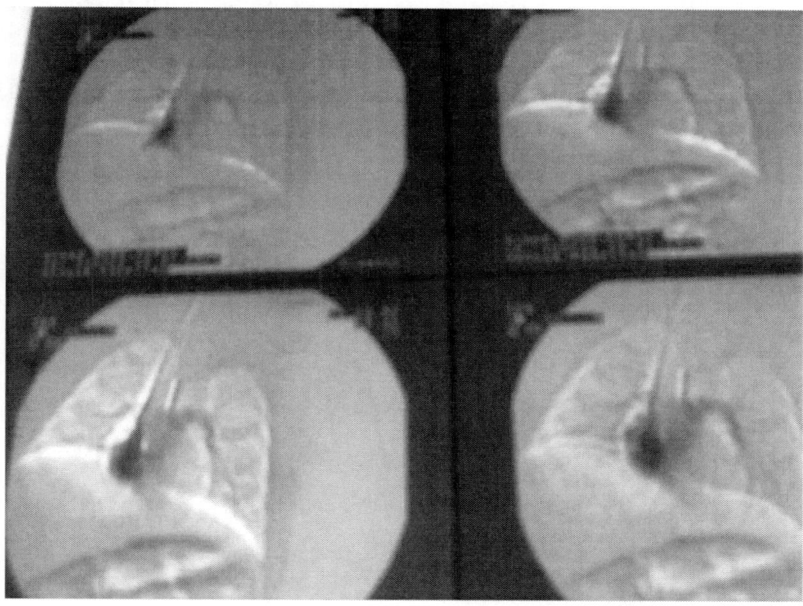

Figure 39. The per-operative films showing contrast injection in the atrial catheter to confirm its position in the right atrium.

IV. Ventriculo-Pleural (V-Pl) Shunts [1-12, 19]

This procedure in under taken only when the abdominal cavity or venous accesses are not available for shunting in neonates, infants and children. The insertion of the ventricular catheter is performed same as in VP shunt through a parietal/frontal burr hole into the lateral ventricle. Then, the shunt chamber is placed either on the burr hole or a little away from it and then connected to the unidirectional valve. The proximal part of the pleural catheter is placed subcutaneously connected to the shunt valve and its distal part with the tip inserted into the pleural cavity from any accessible intercostal space: higher the better (usually the anterior, right 2nd intercostal space).

PRINCIPLES OF SHUNT SURGERY IN HYDROCEPHALUS DUE TO BRAIN TUMORS:

Initially, the headaches are located bifrontally and then become generalized (Figure 40). If acute episodes of transient visual obscuration or severe neck pains occur then the possibility of either transtentorial uncal herniation or a cerebellar tonsillar herniation in the foramen magnum be suspected and the CT/MRI scan is performed immediately.

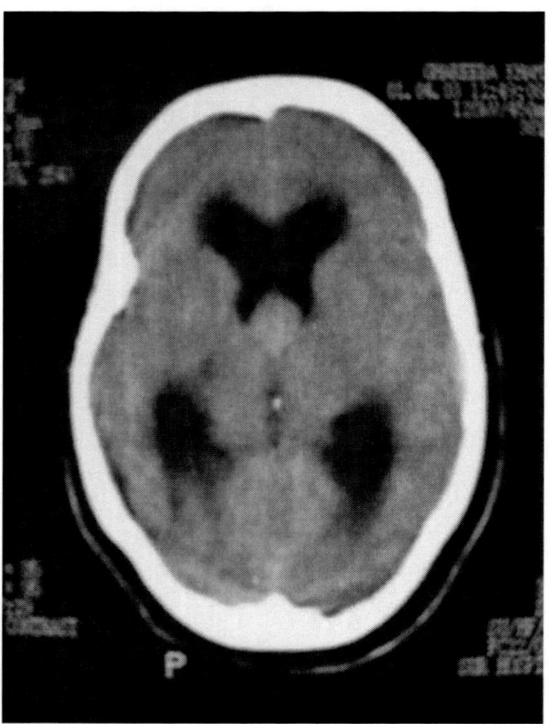

Figure 40. The CT head scan showing a colloid cyst of the anterior third ventricle blocking both the foramen of Monro with bi-ventricular hydrocephalus. This lesion was directly micro-surgically excised and the hydrocephalus was relieved.

The relevant emergent action (ventriculostomy with external ventricular drain or CSF shunting) is taken at that time (as a function as well as life saving procedure) for a better clinical outcome. Then, the causative lesion of the hydrocephalus is surgically dealt with at a later date.

In sub-acute and chronic situations, the important decision is whether to do the CSF shunting first and then excise the causative lesion or vice versa. In modern era of micro-neurosurgery, the benign offending lesion is dealt with first but with a possibility of shunt surgery at a later date.

In cases of significant hydrocephalus due to the malignant lesion in the ventricle, in juxta -ventricular locations or near tentorial hitus/foramen magnum, the author (RR Sharma) usually prefers the CSF shunting as the first procedure followed by the excision of the lesion. Even in cases of significant hydrocephalus due to benign midline skull base tumors such as giant petro-clival meningiomas /chordomas, the CSF shunting as a primary procedure has a significant positive role before excising the lesion per say. However, needless to say, each case is evaluated and treated on its own merits and demerits.

Complications of the Shunt Surgery [42]

Shunt surgery is basically performed to divert the CSF under raised pressure from the cerebral ventricular cavity to extra-ventricular space. Shunt surgery normalizes the CSF pressure for the smooth functioning of the brain and avert high CSF pressure related brain distortions and dysfunctions. The great majority of neurosurgical procedures such as shunt surgery are associated with significant risks of morbidities and mortality. Clinical evaluation with careful history taking and detailed examination is performed. Shunt survey on plain X-rays is performed to determine shunt placement and its continuity. The CT brain scan is done to assess ventricular size, interval enlargement and evidence of pressure effects. The MRI brain scans are helpful in assessing the current state of the cortical-subcortical brain tissues, ventricular anatomy, pathological displacement and distortion of the brain, trans-ependymal seepage of the CSF as well as burr hole -to-ventricle trajectory of the shunt system. Burr hole or Shunt tapping (Figures 41-42) is performed as needed to measure and relieve increased ICP, to sample CSF for exclusion of shunt infection and to confirm the patency of both proximal and distal portions of the shunt. Rarely, the shunt-o-gram is performed to establish shunt patency. Ultrasound study of the abdomen is very useful in assessing the distal shunt malfunction when there are signs of infection and the possibility of pseudo-cyst is high. Interestingly, radio-nuclide shunt flow (isotope study) is measured in NPH where ventricle does not change much. This study helps to establish whether there is any drainage of CSF from the cerebral ventricle to the peritoneal cavity via the shunt system. The CT brain scan and the MRI brain scans are far more informative than any other techniques, as mentioned earlier.

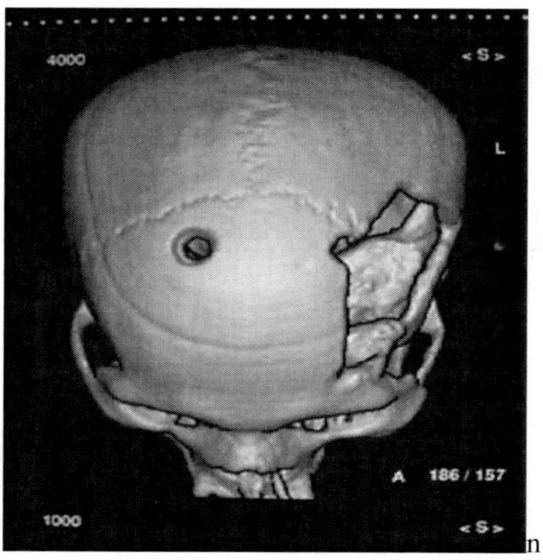

Figure 41. The MIP reconstruction CT Head showing the right frontal burr hole for an emergency tapping of the lateral ventricle (in a case of an operated left frontal EDH with severe head injury) with moderate hydrocephalus.

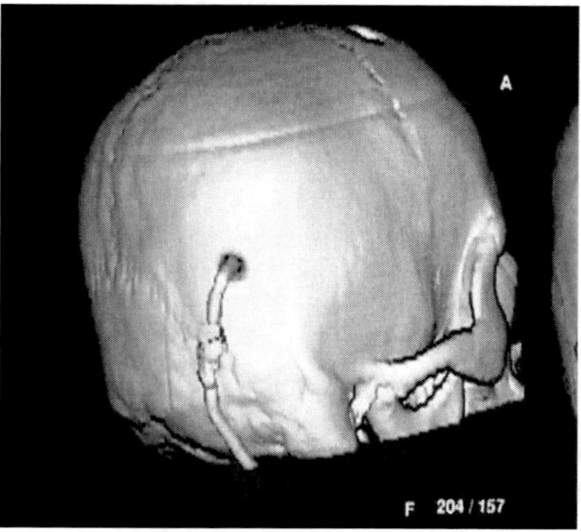

Figure 42. The MIP reconstruction CT HEAD showing the proximal catheter in place at the parietal burr hole and well connected to the valve.

The Classification of the Complications of Shunt Surgery: General versus Specific [43]

The complications common to all shunting procedures are called general (Category I) and the ones which are associated with a particular procedure are called specific (Category II). Category I. The general complications of shunt surgery may be categorized as follows for the sake of simplicity: common, less common, uncommon and rare complications. The common complications are obstruction, infection, hemorrhage, dis-connection, slit ventricle syndrome, and seizures disorders, besides specific complications related to a particular type of shunt surgery. The frequency of common VP shunt complications are as follows: obstruction (15% of all complications; proximal about 80% and distal 20%), infection (10%), hemorrhage (05%), disconnections (05%), slit ventricle (10%), seizures (15%), etc. The less common complications are chronic SDH and Intermittent blockage of the shunt system. The uncommon complications are calcified SDH and the trapped fourth ventricle; the rare complications are cranio-stenosis, micro-cephaly and mortality. Category-II. The complications specific to the type of CSF diversion procedure such as shunt surgery and Neuro-endoscopic third ventriculostomy: VP Shunt, VA shunt,V-PL Shunt, LP shunt, NTV, etc.

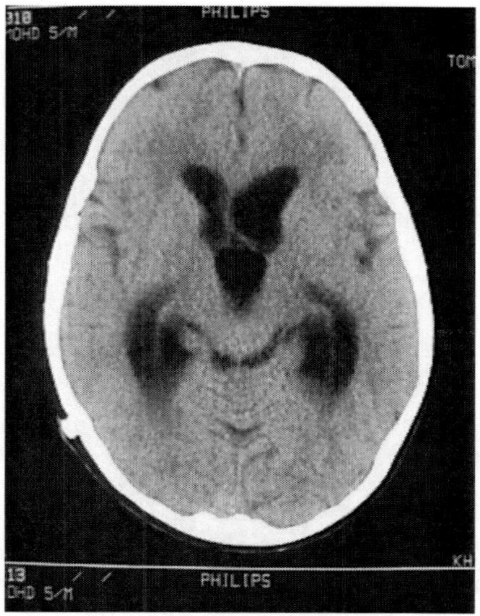

Figure 43. The CT head showing dilated ventricles with peri-ventricular lucencies in a case of right VP shunt.

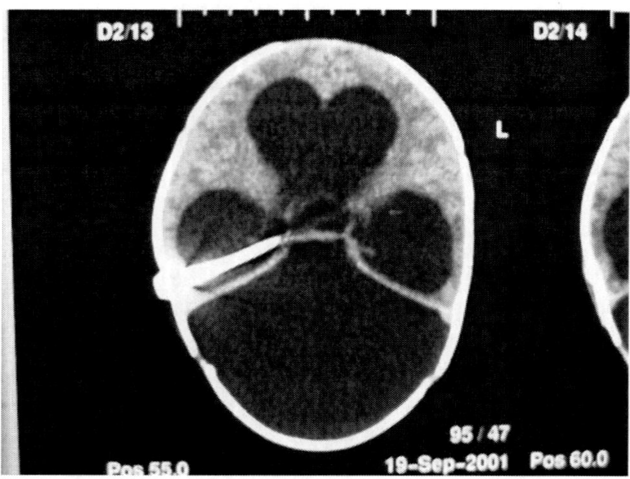

Figure 44. The CT Head showing blocked proximal end with re-expansion of the supratentorial ventricles in a case of extremely severe Dandy-Walker syndrome.

CATEGORY I: GENERAL COMPLICATIONS OF SHUNT SURGERY

Following complications are common to many types of shunting procedures and therefore, these are discussed in some details.

1. Shunt blockage/obstruction. This is by far the most common complication of the shunting procedures. All the components of the shunt system are at risk of obstruction (Figures 41-44).

   A. Proximal shunt block [1-12,39-42] can result simply due to an anchoring stitch tie-blocking the catheter lumen, bleeding, choroid plexus, disconnections, extra-ventricular placement, fluid characteristics(-high CSF protein, cellular debris), and gradual migration of the shunt tube out of the ventricle. The prevention and management of proximal shunt complications are important (Figure 45). These can be achieved by taking simple precautions like by placing the shunt catheter tip anterior to the foramen of Monro to avoid intermingling with the choroid plexus in lateral ventricles; by testing, both, proximal and distal shunt catheters for CSF flow before connecting them; and by being careful when

handling the ventricular catheter which got tangled and stuck choroid plexus. It can be removed with patience by rotational method (Figure 46) and stylet coagulation technique or the removal is performed under direct vision(craniotomy / endoscopic). If there is any higher risk of bleeding then it is better to leave it alone and make a new burr hole for a new catheter. The shunt chamber and the valve are usually blocked with debris, blood, colonization, etc. Once this happens, these components are completely replaced with a new shunt system and all the components are sent for culture and antibiotic sensitivity.

B. Distal shunt obstruction can occur simply a result of progressive shortening of the distal catheter duing the body growth period. There are many other causes of distal shunt block such as blood clot, debries, colonization, infectionand pseudo-cyst (Figures 47-49), omentum entrapment, fracture/disconnection of the catheter, erosion/ perforation of visceral walls (intestine, anus, bladder, vagina, and scrotum), etc.

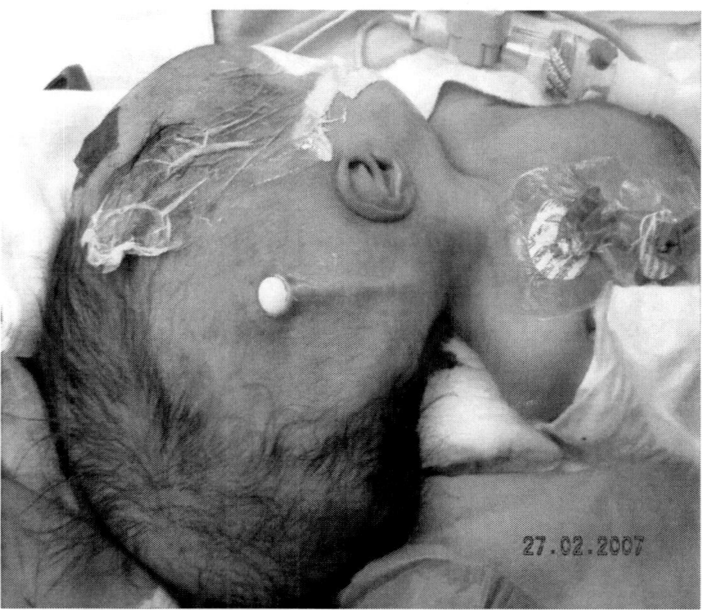

Figure 45. The preventable complication of the shunt surgery: loss of skin overlying the shunt chamber due to continued positioning in a case of congenital hydrocephalus.

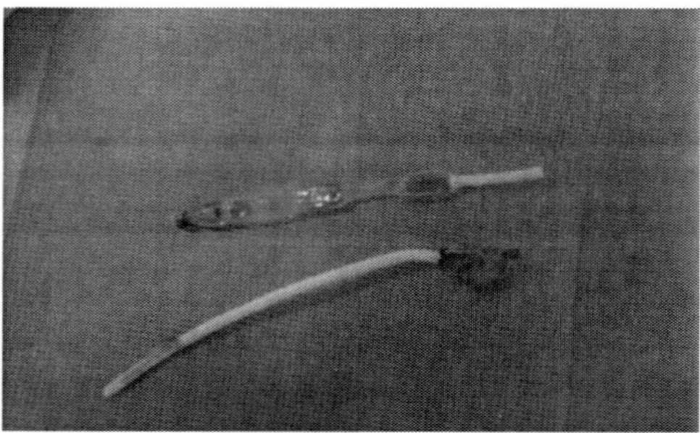

Figure 46. The proximal shunt catheter block due to the choroid plexus entrapment (which was successfully released by the stylet coagulation technique) and the shunt chamber and programable valve blockage due to debris.

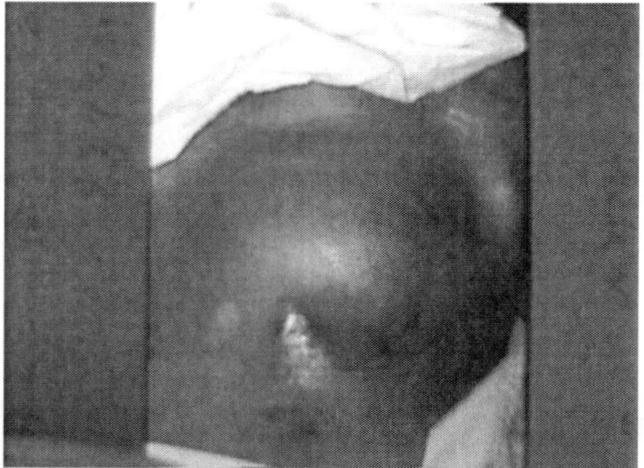

Figure 47. Abdominal swelling in a case of distal shunt catheter block and discovery of a pseudocyst.

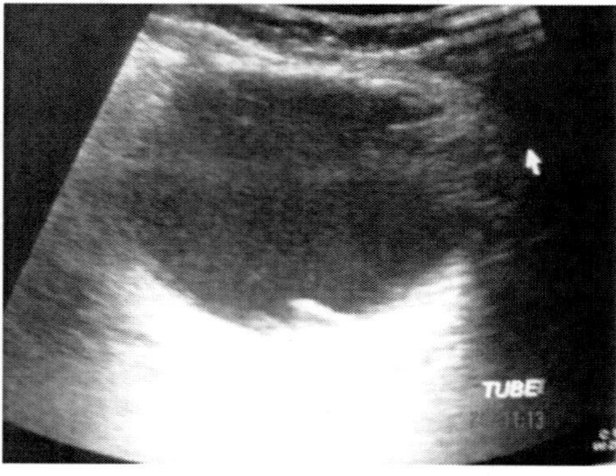

Figure 48. Abdominal ultrasonography showed a localized pseudo-cyst with the tip of the abdominal shunt tube in it.

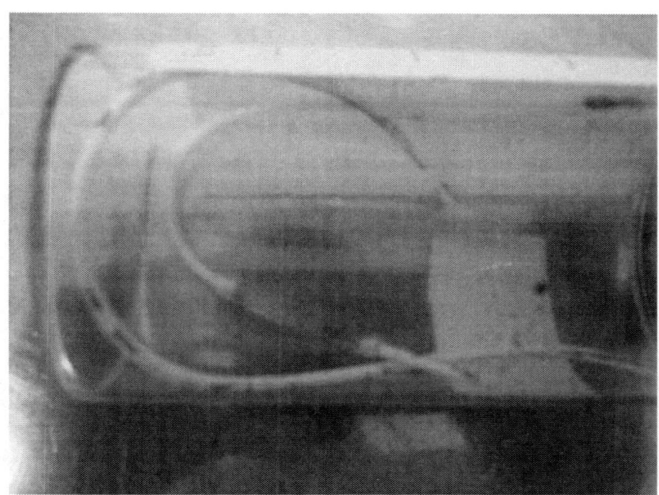

Figure 49. The shunt chamber and the distal shunt cather is blocked with the debris in a case of premature baby with intraventricular hemorrhage.

2. Shunt infection is a formidable cause of shunt morbidities and mortality. [43-46] The incidence of shunt infections is about 2-10 % in first time shunts and 5-15% in multiple revisions. Nearly in about 66-70% cases, the infection occurs in first month after surgery and In about 80% cases occur in first 6 months after the surgery. The common causative pathogens are Staphylococcus epidermidis, Gram-positive bacilli, Haemophilus influenzae, Streptococcus pneumoniae, Entero-bacilli, Corynebacterium parvum, Propionibacterium acnes (Figures 47-51).

The common presentations of shunt infections are as follows

1. Intracranial infections/manifestations: meningitis, ventriculitis and cerebritis
2. Extracranial infections: these are two types

    A. Intra-tubal infections- recurrent blocks/fever/failure to thrive;
    B. Extra-tubal infections- tenderness, redness, fluid collections along the catheter, cellulitis, erosion-loss of skin tissue with exposure of the chamber and the tube

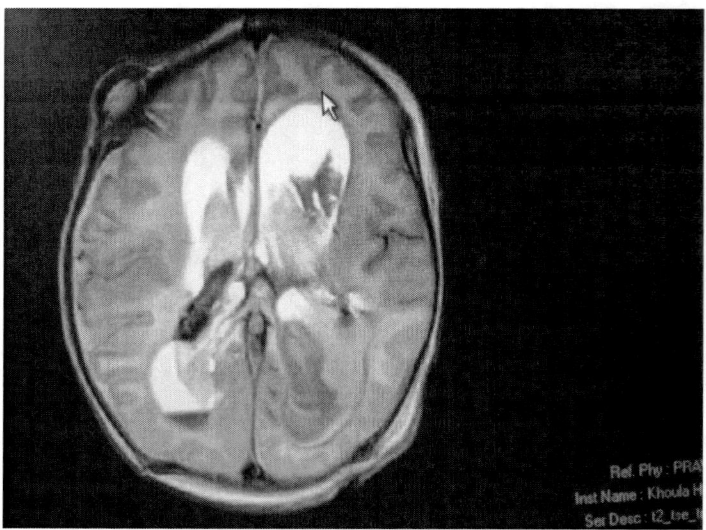

Figure 50. The MRI scan of a meningococcal meningitis patient showing intraventricular hemorrhage, subarachnoid effusions ventriculomegaly and a right frontal sub-galeal reservoir.

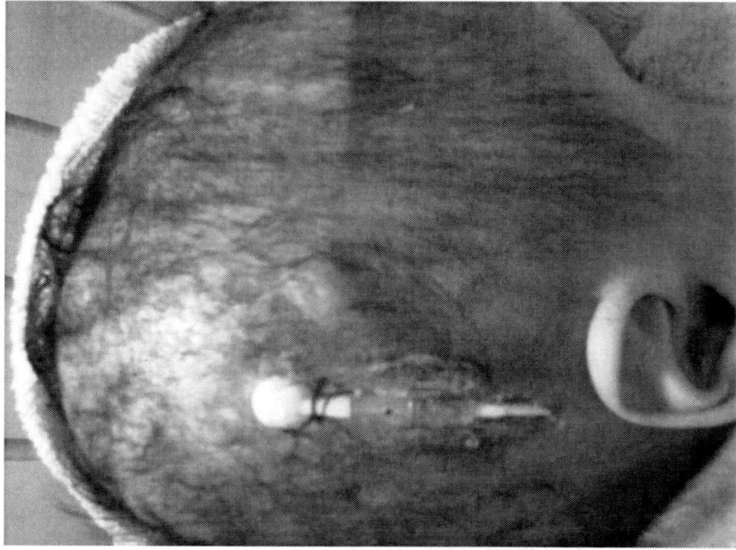

Figure 51. This picture showing the exposed shunt chamber, valve and distal catheter with features of inflammation.

3. Peritoneal infections: localised peritonitis and pseudo-cyst. Shunt infections can also produce obstruction: local peritonitis and pseudo-cyst. In these cases, prolong cultures are needed to detect some resistant species like diphtheroids (7-10 days).

Methods of treating shunt infection vary from institution to institution as no one single method is applicable to all patients. Following are commonly used methods in treating shunt infections:-

A. Antibiotics alone: Both intravenous and in rare instances, intrathecal and intraventricular routes;
B. Antibiotics with shunt removal and delayed re-insertion of the shunt system ;
C. Antibiotics, shunt removal and immediate shunt replacement ;
D. Antibiotics, Shunt removal and external ventricular drainage followed by delayed shunt re-insertion.

Among all the aforementioned tactics, the most logical, successful and predictable management of the shunt infection remains the combination of antibiotics, removal of the infected shunt, external ventricular drain to divert the infected CSF away from the body and insertion of a new shunt system at a different site once the infection is eradicated.

The measures to avoid shunt infection are of paramount important. These, although simple but essential, measures are preoperative antibiotics, special care at the time of aseptic preparation and draping during the surgery, meticulous surgical techniques and handling of the delicate tissues, and vigilant post-operative care.

Shunt nephritis occurs in cases of ventriculo-atrial shunt which present with features of proteinuria, hematuria, and progressive renal failure and this condition is best treated with the removal of shunt. Shunt nephritis is considered to be of diagnostic of shunt infection.

3. Hemorrhage: This is relatively less common complication (Figures 52-53). Usually, there is some bleeding in the subcutaneous tissues when it is tunnelled for placing the distal catheter or there may be some bleeding from the sutured wound edges. However, uncommonly, the bleeding can occur along the trajectory of the proximal shunt catheter: ventricular bleed (IVH), brain tissue (ICH), burr hole site (EDH, SDH, SAH), and subcutaneous scalp hematoma.

As a result of distal catheter placement, it will be very unusual to have intra-peritoneal bleed in the abdomen. The bleeding in various locations along the trajectory of the shunt is best treated as per the clinical manifestation as well as the site and amount of the bleed. The treatment plan is tailored to the needs of an individual patient. However, the prompt management will limit further damage. One of the main concerns is intra-ventricular hemorrhage as it risks shunt blockage and infection. The management aim is to clear the blood from the ventricular system: repeated irrigations, with saline, clear the CSF in majority of cases. However, if the CSF still remains blood-tinged then an external ventricular drain (EVD) is placed till the CSF clears of the blood. When the ventricular CSF is satisfactorily cleared of the blood, then the revision of the shunt is performed.

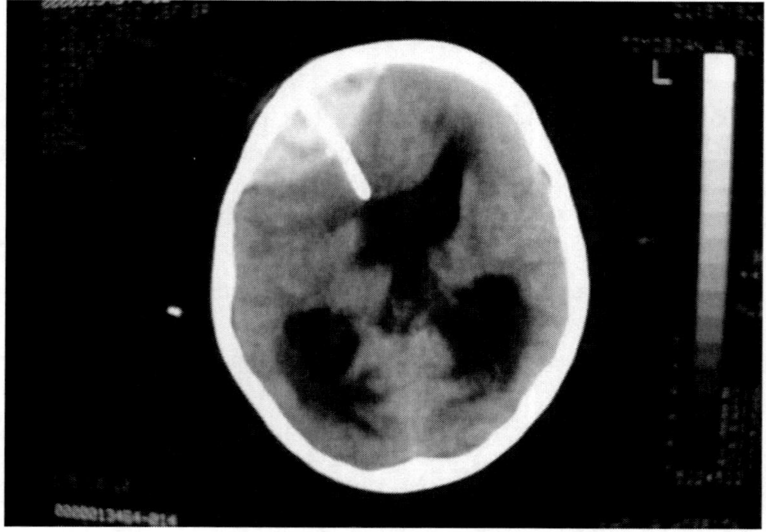

Figure 52. The CT head showing development of the EDH at the site of the proximal catheter placement.

4. Shunt Related Mechanical Complications [39-42]

The shunt being a foreign material, always there is risk of material failure (fracture, dis-connection, erosion and damage), and mechanical effect such as mal-position, migration and perforation of body tissues: brain tissue, scalp, skin, abdominal walls, and organ cavities(intestine, anus, bladder, vagina and scrotum). These cases are treated with removal of the old shunt and insertion of the new one. Other supportive measures are undertaken as needed.

5. Small / Slit Ventricles: [47] This complication is seen less frequently then the shunt obstruction and infection. It poses a great challenge to its management. In an usual scenario, the patient presents with typical symptomatology of shunt blockage and the CT head show small chinked slit ventricles with the presence of the tip of the proximal catheter in one of the slit ventricle along with the compromised supero-lateral cortical sulci as well as basal cisterns. These features are mimicking benign intracranial hypertension. Some of the patient may even settle with acetazolamide, furosemide, etc. But many patients need revision of the shunt. During the revision of the shunt, the CSF flow may be in drops or altogether absent.

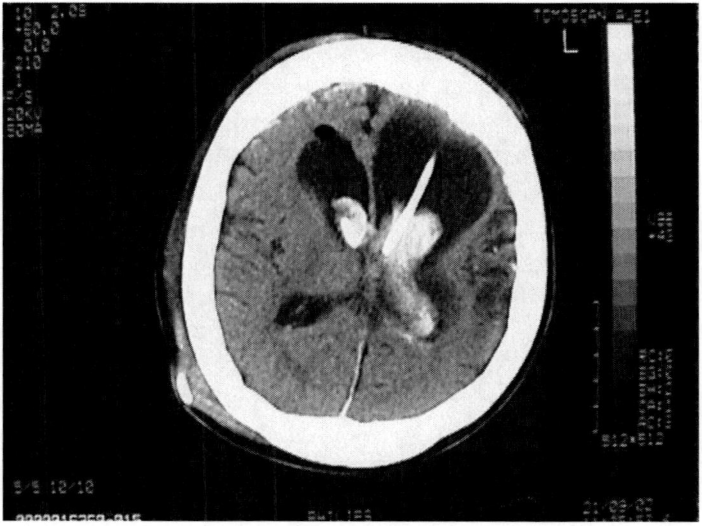

Figure 53. The CT Head showing left frontal catheter in the frontal horn with tri-ventricular bleed and associated hydrocephalus with preserved cerebral sulci.

Initially, the ventricular catheter is flushed with a small amount of saline and if no satisfactory result then it needs to be changed; otherwise, the shunt is reconnected.

When it is decided that the proximal catheter needs replacement, then a great care is exercised in its performance because the ventricles are slit like which poses a great difficulty in their cannulation.

It is better to leave the proximal catheter in its place and insert a new catheter at another (frontal) site. If this does not worked out due to small sized ventricles and then the attempt is made to remove the old catheter and slide a new catheter down the same tract without using a stylet or brain needle because it may veer off the existing tract and miss the ventricle.If the canulation still missed the ventricles then the next option is to try with a brain needle or stylet and if neuro-endoscopy is handy then make a good use of it to place the catheter in the ventricle. Collapsed ventricle itself can occlude the proximal catheter.

If all these maneuvers fail, then it is better to abort the surgery and place the patient in Neuro- ICU for intensive observations with neurological monitoring and recording of ICP. Patient is given mannitol, furosemide, acetazolamide, etc. The serial CT Head scans are performed to regularly check the ventricular size. Once it is apparent that the ventricles are large enough to be catheterized then the re-insertion of the shunt (with a high opening pressure in a programmable shunt system) is done as soon as possible. This will result in a satisfactory outcome. The risks of shunt surgery in this entity are more serious because of the uncertainty of the ventricular cannulation and a non-functioning proximal end. Occasionally, when nothing works, then subtemporal craniectomies with dural dompressions are performed to improve cerebral compliance and to achieve some ventricular dilatation for CSF shunting.

6. Seizures: Epileptic seizures occur in about 10-15% of patients with shunt surgery. These patients, mostly, develop generalized tonic clonic seizures and are assessed with the periodic EEG. They are basically managed with anticonvulsant therapy: monotherapy is preferred over the polytherapy. Sodium valproat, phenytoin sodium, carbamazepine, topiramate, leviteracetam, etc are commonly used and periodically monitored. Patients, who give history of two of more seizures immediately after the shunt surgery only, are treated for a period of 6-9 months. However, patients with continued seizures are treated for a two year fit free period.

CATEGORY II. THE COMPLICATIONS SPECIFIC TO THE TYPE OF SHUNT SURGERY [48]

These are specific complications related to the type of the surgical procedure undertaken: VP Shunt, VA shunt, V-PL Shunt, LP shunt etc. Each procedure is unique in its own rights with its benefits, limitations, morbidities and mortality. Hence, these complications are summarized here. The complications related to the proximal ventricular end are common to most of these shunting surgical procedures and therefore, these were considered in "the Category-I general complications" above.

A. Abdominal complications of VP and LP shunt surgeries: Hydroceles ; migration of the catheter tip in the subcutaneous tissues; penetrating injury to the abdominal viscera(bowel, bladder, vagina); migrating and extruding catheter from the umbilicus, scrotum, anus etc; abdominal infection(acute with peritonitis, sub-acute with bowel /bladder symptoms and chronic-indolent with pseudo-cyst); etc. Each case is treated on its own merit. The management consists of exteriorizing, revising, replacing, re-sitting or re-locating the shunt along with the supportive measures and skillful assistance.
B. Cardiovascular complications of VA shunts: In general, the complications associated with the VA shunt are more frequent and serious than the ventriculo-peritoneal or ventriculo-pleural shunts due mainly to the direct involvement of the cardio-vascular system. Complications of the VA shunt are related to the migration of the catheter tip into the right ventricle of the heart, pulmonary artery or in superior or inferior vena cava; catheter blockage with clot; thrombosis of the venous system with or without pulmonary embolism, pulmonary hypertension, cor-pulmonale; shunt nephritis; septicemia; etc. Rarely, cardiac perforation may occur with tamponade effects and high mortality in such cases. Management, in general, consists of the removal of the VA shunt, intravenous antibiotics, and supportive measures as needed and performance of an alternative CSF diversion procedure.
C. Pleural-pulmonary complications of ventriculo-pleural (V-PL) shunts: Pulmonary/pleural complications of the ventriculo-pleural shunts commonly include mild pneumo-thorax and hemo-thorax and in rare instances, significant pleuritis, pleural effusion and extremely rarely,

the empyema formation may occur. These cases are managed on their own considerations and merits.

D. Lumbar complications of lumbo-peritoneal (LP) shunts : The slippage of the catheter from the lumbar cistern, infection resulting in meningitis and arachnoiditis, CSF leaks, rarely nerve root damage and especially in children the possibilities of scoliosis are the main risks of this technique. Attention to details of the aseptic principles and surgical techniques, minimize these complications. Treatment is tailored to the needs of managing these complications. Reinsertion of the shunt tube, control of the CSF leak, intravenous antibiotics, supportive measures, and physiotherapy for the lower limbs, etc are main therapeutic areas.

E. Intra-cranial complications of neuro-endoscopic third ventriculostomy: [49] The third ventriculostomy is a relatively safe procedure but not without risks. The complications are as follows: Bleeding (Figure-54), infection, diabetes insipidus, hypothalamic damage, vascular injuries (basilar artery), neural injuries (oculo-motor nerve), other morbidities and rarely mortality.

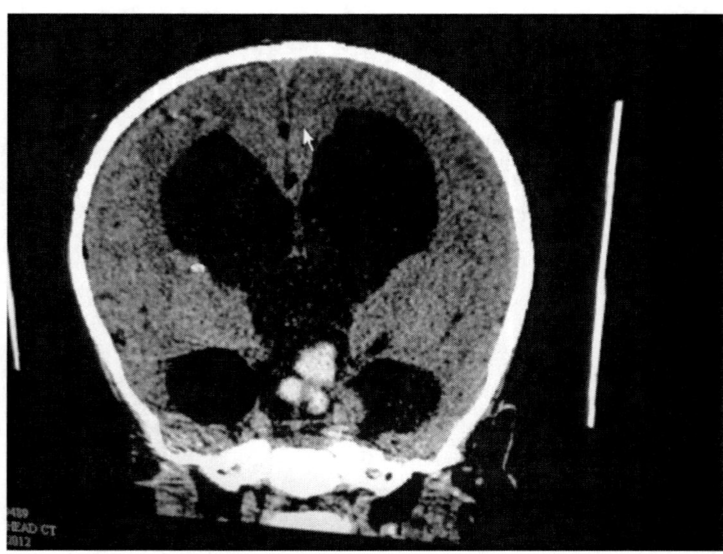

Figure 54. The coronal CT Head scan showing bleeding in the third ventricle following third ventriculostomy: The patient initially worsened in the post operative period and then showed steady improvement but needed a shunt surgery later on.

Conclusion of the CSF Diversion (Shunting and Ventriculostomy) Procedures [50-52]

The shunting and ventriculostomy are the main, two, surgical modalities in neurosurgery to manage the symptomatic patients with communicating and non-communicating hydrocephalus. Attention to details of the surgical procedure is of paramount importance in minimizing the morbidities and mortality associated with these procedures. The prompt recognition and management of the complications associated with these procedures cannot be over emphasized.

Currently, the continuous research is on in many institutions all over the world to find alternatives to the shunt surgery and Neuro- endoscopic third ventriculostomy (NTV), such as by medical means or by the surgical interventions with less morbidities and mortality.

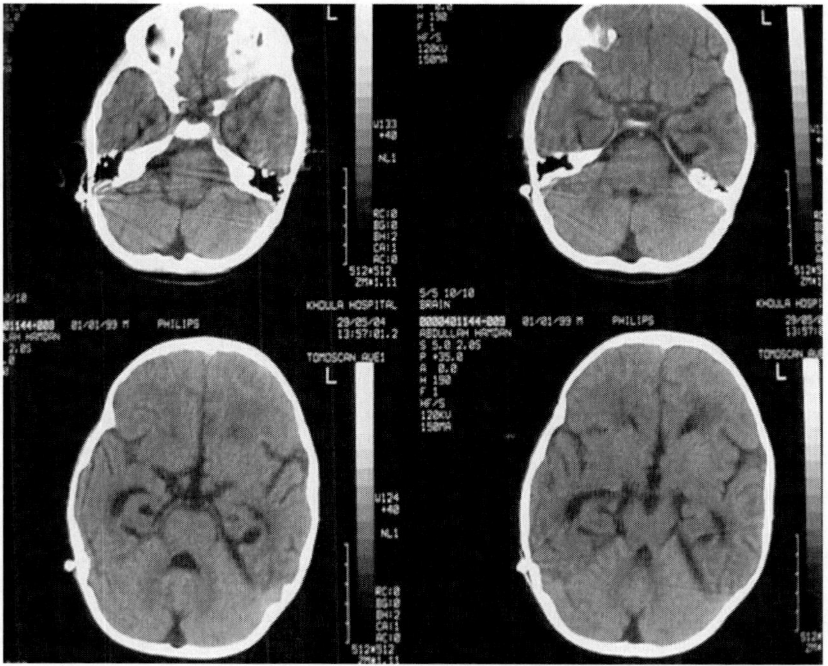

Figures 55. The CT head in a case of right VP Shunt showing a satisfactory intracranial status but the patient was left with impairment of higher mental functions.

Clinical outcome of the management of the hydrocephalus- Hydrocephalus is a clinical manifestation of many diverse disease processes and is not a disease in itself. The extent of the brain damage, due to the effects of the hydrocephalus and its etiology, is the ultimate deciding factor in the overall prognosis of these cases (Figures 55-56). Untreated patients have extremely poor prognosis with large head, thin cerebral parenchyma, and moribund clinical state and largely generate great anxiety and frustration in parents on one side and medical faculty on the other. There is about 50% mortality during infancy and severe intellectual and physical morbidities in 50-60% of the survivors. Whereas, well treated patients have only 10-15 % mortality and 30% intellectual and physical morbidity. Interestingly, more than 50% of such cases achieve normal intelligence. In patients with residual morbidity, lot more depends on the etiology of the hydrocephalus.

Absence of infection, intracranial hemorrhage, trauma, prematurity and congenital malformations (including intrauterine gross hydrocephalus, aqueduct stenosis, Dandy-Walker syndrome, and myelo-dysplasia, etc) favorably affects the prognosis in terms of development of nonverbal and verbal memory as well as motor and visuomotor skills; whereas, their presence, needless to say, adversely affects. Interestingly, even well treated children with hydrocephalus, who appear to have near normal intelligence, still have great learning difficulties as compared to the normal children in the same age groups? These children may have eidetic imagery of the visual or auditory experiences in the past. Many of the children treated for the hydrocephalus associated with spina bifida do not gain normal intelligence. According to Tew and Laurance, these children might have cocktail party syndrome: [50] they can carry on glibly chatty conversations but are unable to get into the real intellectual interactions and discussions. [50-54] Non-verbal intelligence and visuo-motor skills suffer more than the verbal intelligence in many of these children treated for congenital hydrocephalus due to significant thinning of their cerebral mantle and consequent disturbances of the visual, auditory, somato-sensory and motor experiences. In cases of hydrocephalus due to inheritable X-linked aqueductal stenosis, the CSF shunting obviously improves their raised ICP symptoms but usually does not improve their mental retardation.

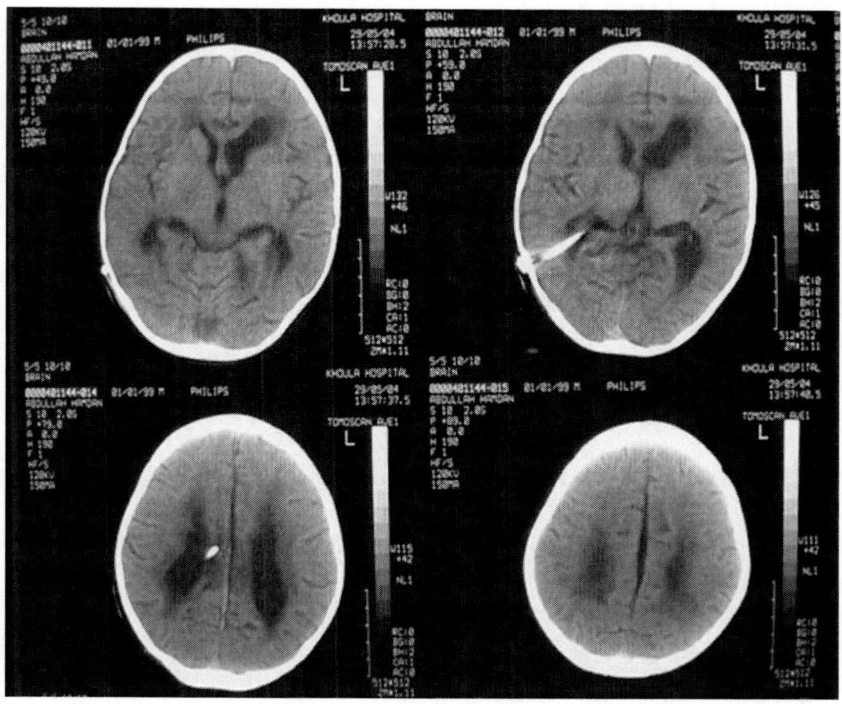

Figure 56. The CT head showing a functioning shunt, with well decompressed ventricles and opened up cerebral sulci and left para-falcine subdural space.

ACKNOWLEDGMENTS

We sincerely thank all the members of the departments of neurosurgery and radiology as well as the nursing staff working in the operation theatres, ICU and the indoor wards for their help and support for these cases. Our especial thanks to Dr Sharif Al Qadi, Specialist Neurosurgeon; Dr Neeraj Salhotra, Senior specialist Neurosurgeon, Dr Said Al Mugherie, Dr Praveen Kharangate, Specialist Neurosurgeon and Dr Najm, specialist Neurosurgeon for the Neuro-imaging pictures and operative photographs.

References

[1] Aschoff A, Kremer P, Hashemi B, Kunze S. The scientific history of hydrocephalus and its treatment. *Neurosurg. Rev.*1999;22:67-95.

[2] Jea A, Al Otibi M, Bonnard A, Drake JM. Laproscopic-assisted ventriculoperitoneal shunt surgery in children:a series of 11 cases. *J. Neurosurg.* 2007;106(6 suppl):421-425.

[3] Pudenz RH. The surgical treatment of hydrocephalus—a historical review. *Surg. Neurol.*1980;15:15-26.

[4] Pawar SJ, Sharma RR, Mahapatra AK, Lad SD. 'Intracranial Pressure Monitoring in severe head injury'. Illustrated Synopsis- Head injury conference, Oman. Al Zahra Printers, Oman, April, 2000. PP 72-76.

[5] Meier U, Zeilinger FS, Kintzel D. Signs, symptoms and course of normal pressure hydrocephalus in comparison with cerebral atrophy. *Acta Neurochir.* 1999;141:1039-1048.

[6] Sharma RR. Fungal infections of the nervous system:Current perspective and controversies in their management. *International Journal of Surgery* 8 (2010) :591-601.

[7] Sharma RR, Pawar SJ, Lad SD, Mishra GP, Netalkar AS. Rege S. Fungal infections of the central nervous system. In Schmidek and Sweet Operative Neurosurgical Techniques: Indications, Methods, and Results.6e, Vol.2, Chapter 149, Alfredo Quinones-Hinojosa(ed).2012, Elsevier Inc, Saunders, Phladelphia, USA.pp 1691-1732.

[8] Prabhu SS, Sharma RR, Gurusinghe NT, Parekh HC. Acute transient hydrocephalus in carbon monoxide poisoning. A case report. *J. Neurol. Neurosurg. Psychiatry,* 1993; 56:567-568.

[9] Sharma RR, Chandy MJ, Lad SD. Transient hydrocephalus and acute lead encephalopathy in neonates and infants. Report of two cases. *British Journal of Neurosurgery*, 1990; 4: 141-146.

[10] Sharma RR, Sharma Apollina, Raniga S. Current concepts of meningitis: Its etiological factors, management options and prognosis.In, Text book:Meningitis, Causes, Diagnosis and Treatment: Grogoris Houllis and Magalini Karachalios (editors), Series:Neuroscience research progress. Nova Publishers, New York, USA, March2012. PP. 1-82.

[11] Rodrigues D, Mahapatra AK, Sharma RR, Lad SD, Pawar SJ. Post traumatic hydrocephalus. In: Sharma RR, Pawar SJ, Lad SD (eds). Illustrated Synopsis: Management of Head Injury in Oman. Al Zahra Printers, Muscat Oman, April 2000, pp 100-102.

[12] Rodrigues D, Sharma RR, Sousa J, Pawar SJ. Post traumatic hydrocephalus in severe head injury- a study of 22 cases. - *The Pan Arab Journal of Neurosurgery*; 2000, 4(2): 63-67.

[13] Sharma RR, Chandy MJ, Lad SD. Colloid cyst of the third ventricle complicating pregnancy. Case report and review of literature. *Annals of Saudi Medicine* 1990; 10(4) : 457-459.

[14] Venkitaramanan CS, Sharma RR, Lad SD, Chandy MJ. Role of shunt surgery in vertebro-basilar infarcts and obstructive hydrocephalus. *Medical Newsletter* (Oman) 1990; (1) 19-22.

[15] Shapiro, K, Fried A.: Pressure-volume relationships in shunt dependent childhood hydrocephalus. The zone of pressure instability in children with acute deterioration. *J. Neurosurgery*., 64:390-396,1986.

[16] Shapiro K, Fried A, Marmarou A.: Biomechanical and hydrodynamic characterization of the hydrocephalic infant. *J. Neurosurg.* 63:69-75,1985.

[17] Sharma RR, Chandy MJ, Shunt surgery in growing skull fractures. Report of two cases. *British Journal of Neurosurgery*. 1991; 5, 93-98.

[18] Frim DM, Penn R, Lacy M. Surgical management of hydrocephalus. In Schmidek and Sweet Operative Neurosurgical Techniques: Indications, Methods, and Results.6e, Vol.1, Chapter 94, Alfredo Quinones-Hinojosa(ed).2012, Elsevier Inc, Saunders, Phladelphia, USA. Pp 1127-1134.

[19] Tew B, Laurence KM: The clinical and psychological characteristics of children with the "cocktail party" syndrome. Z. Kindererchir.Grenzgeb., 28:360-367, 1979.

[20] Young, H., Nulsen, F., Weiss,m., et al.: The relationship of intelligence and cerebral mantle in treated infantile hydrocephalus. *Padiatrics*, 52:38-44,1973.

[21] David C Mc Cullough. Hydrocephalus: Treatment. In Wilkins RH, Rengachary SS (eds). Neurosurgery. Vol.3, McGraw Hill Book Company, New York,1985.

[22] Jea A, Al Otibi M, Rutka JT, Dirks PB, Kulkarni AV, Taylor MD, et al. The history of neurosurgery at the hospital for sick children in Toronto. *Neurosurgery*.2007;61(3):612-624.

[23] Yampolsky C, Ajler P. Management of shunt infections. In Schmidek and Sweet Operative Neurosurgical Techniques: Indications, Methods, and Results.6e, Vol.1, Chapter 94, Alfredo Quinones-Hinojosa(ed).2012, Elsevier Inc, Saunders, Phladelphia, USA. Pp 1151-1157.

[24] Shinnar S, Gammon K, Bergman EW Jr., et al.: Management of hydrocephalus in infancy: Use of acetazolamide and furosemide to avoid cerebrospinal shunts. *J. Pediatr.*, 107:31-37,1985.

[25] Abbott R. History of neuroendoscopy. *Neurosurg. Clin. North Am.* 2004;15:1-7.

[26] Dandy WE. An operative procedure for hydrocephalus. *Bull. Johns Hopkins Hosp.* 1922;33:89-90.

[27] Grant JA. Victor Darwin Lespinasse: a biographical sketch. *Neurosurgery.* 1996; 39:1232-1233.

[28] Dandy W. Extirpation of the choroid plexus of the lateral ventricles in communicating hydrocephalus. *Ann. Surg.*1918; 68:569.

[29] Mixter WJ. Ventriculoscopy and puncture of the third ventricle. *Boston Medical and surgical Journal.* 1923; 188:277-278.

[30] Goumnerova LC, FRIM DM. Treatment of hydrocephalus with third ventrivulocisternostomy: outcome and CSF flow patterns. *Pediatr. Neurosurg.* 1997; 27:-149-152.

[31] Li KW, Nelson C, Suk I, Jalo GI. Neuroendoscopy:past, present, and future. *Neurosurgical focus.*2005; 19:E1.

[32] Di Rocco F, Grevent D, Drake JM, Boddaert N, Puget S, Roujeau T, Blauwblomme T, Zerah M, Brunelle F, Sainte-Rose C. Changes in intracranial CSF distribution after ETV.In: Recinos PF, Jallo GI, Recinos VR. Endoscopic third ventriculostomy. In Schmidek and Sweet Operative Neurosurgical Techniques: Indications, Methods, and Results. 6e, Vol.1, Chapter 94, Alfredo Quinones-Hinojosa(ed).2012, Elsevier Inc, Saunders, Phladelphia, USA. Pp 1143-1150.

[33] *Childs Nerv Syst.* 2012 Jul; 28(7):997-1002.

[34] Drake J, Chumas P, Kestle J, et al. Late rapid deterioration after endoscopic third ventriculostomy: additional cases and review of the literature. *J. Neurosurg.* 2006 Aug; 105(2 suppl):118-126.

[35] King JA, Auguste KI, Halliday W, Drake JM, Kulkarni, AV. Ventriculocystostomy and endoscopic third ventriculostomy/shunt placement in the management of hydrocephalus secondary to giant retrocerebellar cysts in infancy. *J. Neurosurg. Pediatr.* 2010;5:403-407.

[36] Kulkarni AV, Drake JM, Mallucci CL, et al. Endoscopic third ventriculostomy in the treatment of childhood hydrocephalus. *J. Pediatr.* 2009; 155:254-259:e251.

[37] Scarff J. Endoscopic treatment of hydrocephalus: description of a ventriculoscope and a preliminary report of cases. *Arch. Neurol. Psychiatry.*1936; 35:853.

[38] Warf BC, Kulkarni A. Intraoperative assessment of cerebral aqueduct patency and cisternal scarring: impact on success of endoscopic third ventriculostomy in 403 African children. *J. Neurosurg. Pediatrics.* 2010;5:204-209.

[39] Drake JM, Singhal A, Kulkarni AV, DeVeber G, Cochrane DD; Canadian Pediatric Neurosurgery Study Group. Consensus definitions of complications for accurate recording and comparisons of surgical outcomes in pediatric neurosurgery. *J. Neurosurg. Pediatr.* 2012 Aug;10(2):89-95.

[40] Drake JM, Kestle John RW, Milner R, et al. Randomised Trial of Cerebrospinal fluid Shunt Valve Design in Pediatric Hydrocephalus. *Neurosurgery.*1998; 43(2):294-303.

[41] Sharma RR, Pawar SJ, Devadas R.V, Dev E.J. 'CT Stereotactic guided lateral trans-cerebellar programmable fourth ventriculo-peritoneal shunting for symptomatic trapped fourth ventricle'. *Clinical Neurology Neurosurgery* 2001; 103:143-146.

[42] Le H, Yamini B, Frim DM. Lumboperitoneal shunting as a treatment for slit ventricle syndrome. *Pediatr. Neurosurg.*2002; 36:178-182.

[43] Wu Y, Green N, Wrensh M,et al. Vetriculoperitoneal shunt complications in California:1990-2000. *Neurosurgery* 2007; 61:557-563.

[44] Borgbjerg BM, Gjerris, Albeck MJ, Borgesen SE. Risk of infection after cerebrospinal fluid shunt: an analusis of 884 first time shunts. *Acta Neurochir.* 1995; 136:1-7.

[45] Gupta S, Vachhrajani S, Kulkarni AV, Taylor MD, et al. Neurosurgical management of extraaxial central nervous system infections in children. *J. Neurosurg. Pediatr.* 2011;7(5):441-451.

[46] James HE, Walsh JW, Wilson HD, et al. The management of CSF shunt infection: a clinical experience. *Acta Neurochir.* (Wien).1981;50:157-166.

[47] Wu Y, Green N, Wrensh M, et al. Vetriculoperitoneal shunt complications in California:1990-2000. Neurosurgery 2007;61:557-563.

[48] Bruce DA, Weprin B. The slit ventricle syndrome. *Neurosurg. Clin. N. Am.* 2001; 12:709-717G.

[49] Al Hinai QS, Pawar SJ, Sharma RR, Devadas RV. Subgaleal migration od a ventriculoperitoneal shunt. *Journal of Clinical Neurosciences.* 2006;13: 666-669.

[50] Recinos PF, Jallo GI, Recinos VR. Endoscopic third ventriculostomy. In Schmidek and Sweet Operative Neurosurgical Techniques: Indications, Methods, and Results. 6e, Vol.1, Chapter 94, Alfredo Quinones-

Hinojosa(ed).2012, Elsevier Inc, Saunders, Phladelphia, USA. Pp 1143-1150.

[51] Tew B, Laurence KM: The clinical and psychological characteristics of children with the "cocktail party" syndrome. Z. Kindererchir.Grenzgeb., 28:360-367, 1979.

[52] Bret P, Guyotat J, Chazal J.Is normal pressure hydrocephalus a valid concept in 2002? A reappraisal in, symptoms five questions and proposal for a new designation of the syndrome as "chronic hydrocephalus." *J. Neurol. Neurosurg. Psychiatry,* 2002; 73:9-12.

[53] Brown E, Edwards R, Pople I. Conservative management of patients with cerebrospinal fluid shunt infections. *Neurosurgery*.2006;58:657-665.

[54] Hebb AO, Cusimano MD. Idiopathic normal pressure hydrocephalus:a systematic review of diagnosis and outcome. *Neurosurgery*. 2001; 49: 1166-1184.

[55] Johnson MC, Maxwell MS. Delayed intrapleural migration of a VP shunt. *Childs Nerv. System,* 1995; 11:348-350.

In: Hydrocephalus
Editor: Amaya Velazquez
ISBN: 978-1-62100-453-0

Chapter 2

CLINICAL FEATURES AND MANAGEMENT

***Se Youn Jang*[1] *and Choong Hyun Kim*[2]**
[1]Department of Neurosurgery, Seoul Medical Center, Seoul, Korea
[2]Department of Neurosurgery, Hanyang University Guri Hospital, Guri, Korea

ABSTRACT

The symptoms of hydrocephalus are developed by the increased intracranial pressure. The main symptoms observed among children include poor feeding, excessive sleepiness, enlarging head with soft areas on the fontanelles, an inability to move eyes upward, and vomiting. Commonly observed symptoms among adults include headache, nausea, ataxia, and visual disturbances. Generally, the earliest and most prominent symptoms of hydrocephalus are balance and gait disturbances. Furthermore, impairment of memory and urgency incontinence is common.

The goal of the treatment for hydrocephalus is to protect the periventricular tissues from pressure and osmotic loads. In order to do so, the intracranial pressure needs to be reduced by decreasing the cerebrospinal fluid (CSF) volume. The medical treatment is decreasing CSF secretion by the choroid plexus-acetazolamide and furosemide and increasing CSF reabsorption-isosorbide. However, surgical CSF diversion is mostly performed. Among the surgical interventions, ventriculoperitoneal (VP) shunt is most commonly used, and, recently, neuroendoscopic techniques are utilized to treat obstructive hydrocephalus.

Hydrocephalus can cause some complications, or complications may develop as a result of the surgery used to treat it. The potential complications of hydrocephalus include cerebral atrophy, neurological deficits, cerebral ischemia, and dementia. The complications of shunt are malfunctions, blockages, and infections.

Keywords: hydrocephalus, symptoms, treatment, complications

Clinical Features

Infants

For infants, hydrocephalus is suspected if the head size increases abnormally. If head circumference is larger than 2 standard deviations compared to the age group, the head size becomes larger than the face, the anterior fontanel is expanded, and the scalp becomes thinner. The increased intracranial pressure causes intracranial blood to flow backward, expanding the vein on the forehead. Eyeballs deviate downward to cover eyelids; there is paralysis of upward gaze, and the sclera above the iris only is visible. This is the so-called setting-sun sign, and convergent strabismus is caused by abducens palsy. It is caused by the compression on the mesencephalic tegmentum by hydrocephalic pressure. A suture diastasis is also shown or felt with fingers.

Moreover, the spastic paralysis including optic nerve atrophy and movement disorder may appear. The posture of infants appears to be gradually flexed arms and legs. This is usually caused by corticospinal track damage. If the head is large and the fontanel is expanded, cracked pot sound is heard by percussion (Macewen's sign). If the head size enlarges progressively, a neuroradiological examination is required for the differential diagnosis of hydrocephalus and other causes.

Children Older than Two Years Old

The head circumference of children older than two years old may be within normal range. However, symptoms including headache, vomiting, visual disturbance, behavioral disorders, memory impairment, poor intelligence, cranial nerve palsies and spastic paralysis in the lower limbs may develop. In severe cases, gait disturbance may occur. Endocrine symptoms such as dwarfism, obesity or a precocious or delayed puberty may appear rarely. The cause for this appearance is compression of hypothalamus or the pituitary stalk by the expanded third ventricles.

Adults

The adult type is different from that of the child based on features of skull growth and its structure. A high-pressure hydrocephalus is often accompanied with bleeding in the subarachnoid space or the meningitis, within a several weeks after such disorder's occurrence, hydrocephalus may occur. After completion of the skull growth, macrocephaly does not occur, while headache, nausea, vomiting, gait disturbance, trunk ataxia, visual disturbance or other may occur from the intracranial pressure increase. In early stages, the headache occurs on both forehead areas. Because drainage of cerebrospinal fluid is not fluent during sleep, the headache becomes more severe in the morning. As the symptom progresses, the headache progresses to the entire head and becomes continuous. Sometimes, nausea and vomiting may accompany the headache. However, the symptoms are not aggravated by head movement in general. Visual loss, a diplopia due to sixth cranial nerve weakness and upward gaze palsy occur, indicating severe damage in the optic nerve due to progression of the intracranial pressure. In this case, a papilledema can be found in a fundoscopic examination.

Normal Pressure Hydrocephalus

A clinical triad is characteristic of normal pressure hydrocephalus. This is a progressive gait disturbance, a memory loss, and incontinence. The gait disturbance is usually the earliest feature, followed by memory loss, and urinary incontinence, lastly.

The gait disturbance is most often the initial feature and occurs in almost 90% of patients. Common symptoms of gait disturbance are unsteadiness, reduced walking speed, impairment of balance, with difficulty encountered on stairs. The gait disturbance in normal pressure hydrocephalus is often confused with Parkinson's Disease, like forward-leaning posture, imbalance exacerbated by eye closure, short steps and stooped gait, but there is no tremor, slowness of alternating movement, mask-like face and lead-pipe rigidity. If hydrocephalus is untreated, the steps may shorten with recurrent falls. Eventually initiating gait, standing, sitting, and balance on turning will be impossible. Urinary symptoms seem to be initially urgency and frequency rather than true incontinence. These symptoms are caused by the involvement of the sacral fibers in the corticospinal tract [5]. Later, the urgency is associated with incontinence, and ultimately there is "frontal lobe incontinence" in which the patient is indifferent to his lapses of continence. Cognitive impairments that we have encountered have been dullness in thinking and action, memory loss, apathy, and slight inattention. The pattern appears to be a frontal subcortical syndrome. Speech disturbance due to motivational problems differs from the cortical deficits of aphasia, apraxia, and agnosia seen in patients with Alzheimer's disease [4,31]. Cognitive impairment in normal pressure hydrocephalus is differentiated from cerebrovascular disease, stroke, Binswanger's disease, Parkinson's disease, Alzheimer's disease, and corticobasal degeneration.

The progression or the expression speed varies, and in certain cases, the symptom occurs after several months or years after appearance of the cause factors. Headache and papilledema are usually not found, but aggressive behavior or seizure and Parkinsonism may appear. No impairment on extraocular muscles is found. Motor paralysis or loss of sense does not exist, if there was no brain damage related to a disease causing the hydrocephalus. This condition often occurs after subarachnoid hemorrhage or meningitis. If the cause is not clear, differentiation from Alzheimer's disease and other diseases with expanded ventricles under normal cerebrospinal fluid pressures are required.

Management

The Principle of Hydrocephalus Management

Since continuous and progressing brain compression is occurring caused by expansion of the ventricle in the hydrocephalus, the diagnosis and the treatment should be made as early as possible before irreversible brain changes. If the ventricle is gradually expanding along with the symptom of intracranial pressure, surgery is typically required. For infants, if thickness of the cerebrum is less than 3.5 cm, surgery within five months after the birth is desirable. And, for a child less than three years old, expression of the symptoms is not easy and evaluation of symptoms is very difficult because adequate tests regarding intelligence and its development are not available; so surgery may be required if the ventricle is expanded. If an adult or a teenager with an enlarged ventricle does not show the intracranial pressure increase, an operative treatment should be carefully made while considering compensatory hydrocephalus and stopped hydrocephalus. If any causes for the hydrocephalus exist, the operation to remove causes should be performed initially.

Temporary Management

1. Medical Treatment

Although the surgical treatment is the ultimate method, administration of 100 mg/kg of Acetazolamide (Diamox®) or 1mg/kg of furosemide to reduce the cerebrospinal fluid creation in the choroid plexus or use of a medicine such as isosorbide to increase the cerebrospinal fluid absorption can be considered. By blocking carbonic anhydrase activity, acetazolamide can decrease CSF production by nearly 100%. Similar results are archived with furosemide [12]. However, as intracranial pressure does not reduce with a medication treatment, the method is not suitable for a long-term treatment. Acetazolamide therapy may slow the rate of ventricular hemorrhage, but long-term use is limited by acidosis and possible myelin toxicity, and metabolic alkalosis and nephrocalcinosis may result from chronic furosemide use [38]. Therefore, no alternative treatment replacing surgery is known yet.

2. Cerebrospinal Fluid Drainage Method

Sometimes, external drainage of cerebrospinal fluid using ventricular puncture or periodic lumbar puncture is helpful. Such methods to control the hydrocephalus temporarily may be used efficiently for hydrocephalus after an intracranial hemorrhage or a post-hemorrhagic hydrocephalus and allows delaying surgery for the case with severe hydrocephalus.

Surgical Management

The first surgical treatment reported in the main literature was performed in Greece by Hippocrates, in the 5th century B.C., who punctured the lateral ventricle in a patient with obstructive hydrocephalus. In the modern era, Lespinasse was the first to make a choroid plexectomy endoscopically, at the beginning of the 20th century, followed by Scarff, who performed the first ventriculostomy on the third ventricular floor [23].

Two main forms of surgical management for hydrocephalus are shunt insertion and endoscopic third ventriculostomy. The most frequently used treatment for the hydrocephalus is the shunt surgery. It makes a bypass to drain the cerebrospinal fluid from the ventricle to other body areas.

1. The Composition and the Principles of the Shunt Device

The shunt device is composed of the proximal catheter, a valve to limit cerebrospinal fluid to flow only one direction, and the distal catheter. The ideal placement of the proximal catheter avoids areas of functional neuroanatomy and the choroid plexus while being at sufficient depth for cerebrospinal fluid drainage to occur through all distal drainage openings despite changes in ventricular size. In the shunt device, the drainage level of cerebrospinal fluid is defined with the difference of pressure caused by the internal pressure of the ventricle, the valve's resistance and the high differences between the proximal catheter and the distal catheter. Therefore, if the intracranial pressure is too high, or if a tall man is standing up, a siphon phenomenon due to increased cerebrospinal fluid pressure difference proportional to the increased vertical distance between height of the head (proximal catheter) and the abdominal cavity occurs. And, due to the siphon phenomenon, the intracranial pressure rapidly declines and may result in complications including a headache or an intracranial hemorrhage. So the valve that can adjust the drainage pressure or the one with siphon prevention device is used for prevention of excessive CSF drainage. Before a shunt operation, the right side of the head skin, the neck, the chest and the abdomen should be well sterilized, and prophylactic antibiotics are administered to reduce infection risks after the operation. It is important to correct the patient's body position to prevent any unnecessary skin incision on the neck or other area.

2. Types of Shunts

2.1. Ventriculo-peritoneal Shunt

This is the most frequently used shunt method, with which the cerebrospinal fluid is drained though the proximal catheter inserted to the lateral ventricle and the valve and passing the hypodermic tissue to the distal catheter inserted to the abdominal cavity. Catheter placement into the peritoneal cavity has many advantages over pleural or vascular sites [18]. The abdomen has a vast absorption capacity and can accept sufficient catheter length to accommodate a lifetime of body growth: tubing mobility minimizes the potential of distal obstruction.

2.2. Lumbo-peritoneal Shunt

This method is to drain the cerebrospinal fluid from lumbar subarachnoid space, which inserts the proximal catheter to the abdominal cavity through the distal catheter. Orin reported that lumbo-peritoneal shunt did not induce over drainage resulting in symptomatic subdural hematoma, which is an intermittent problem with ventriculo-peritoneal shunting. Lumbo-peritoneal shunting should be considered a practical alternative to ventriculo-peritoneal shunting for normal pressure hydrocephalus, especially in high-risk patients or patients who are averse to an intracranial procedure [2]. The lumbo-peritoneal shunt is only applicable for communicating hydrocephalus. If the indication is incorrect and the method is applied, the tonsillar herniation, subdural hematoma or acquired Arnold-Chiari malformation may occur.

2.3. Ventriculo-atrial Shunt

The cerebrospinal fluid is drained through the jugular vein and right atrium. This method is often applied only when the shunt between the ventricle and the abdominal cavity is complicated due to a previous abdominal surgery or a disease in the abdominal cavity, such as peritonitis.

2.4. Patient Care after Shunt Operation

A patient's care after a shunt operation should be performed with the following two objectives: First, a complete skin closure should be performed. It is essential to prevent direct pressure to the valve system for avoidance of any skin problems causing the shunt infection. Secondly, the assessment of shunt function and early detection of shunt complications are important. In general, after a shunt operation, the inserted valve and catheters are checked with a simple x-ray and, after three months, the follow-up check is performed using a computer tomography scan or a magnetic resonance imaging.

Endoscopic Third Ventriculostomy (ETV)

Shunting is generally a successful endeavor, but the constant need for maintenance of malfunctioning shunts, coupled with major technological advances in the field of endoscopic surgery, prompted a renewed interest in third ventriculostomy as a means of managing hydrocephalus [27]. ETV, which makes a hole in the third ventricle floor to pass through the basal cistern, is alternative to the shunt surgery.

It is an established treatment for hydrocephalus, especially since there is no need to place a foreign body such as a ventricular shunt, with its associated possibility of shunt malfunction and/or shunt over drainage [25,30], while the physiological flow of the cerebrospinal fluid is recovered because of the subarachnoid space and the penetration of the third ventricle. Controversy persists over the selection of candidates for ETV, which affects the overall success rate of the procedure [7,10,22,26]. However, the overall success rate of ETV lies somewhere between 50% and 90% at one year [15,24,36] and success rate of 88% with hydrocephalus secondary to tectal glioma [15], but 0% to 33% in patients with intraventricular hemorrhage associated with prematurity [6,33]. So the selection of patients is the key to achieve clinical success in maximizing the chance of success and minimizing the complication in ETV.

Unlike the shunt, the operation is a relatively safe method with no mechanical complication due to the fact that there is no foreign body insertion or no overdrainage or complication with infections while the physiological flow of the cerebrospinal fluid is recovered because of the subarachnoid space and the penetration of the third ventricle. This is known to be efficient in patients with non-communicating (closed) hydrocephalus and normal absorption to the venous system. The treatment is especially effective in recent closed hydrocephalus with a less-than one-year-old baby with no subarachnoid hemorrhage but with the ventricle expansion and the normal anatomical ventricle.

Surgical technique: In the operating room, the patient is positioned with supine position under general endotracheal anesthesia. The puncture is drilled on the front part of coronal suture (3 cm right from the center line of the front part of the coronal suture), and the gray venula removed. After the ventricle is punctured, the cerebrospinal fluid spurts due to the high internal pressure of the ventricle. Along the peel away sheath (14 Fr), a 2 mm endoscope is inserted in the ventricle to check choroid plexus, septal vein, thalamostriate vein, septum pellucidum, caudate nucleus head or bleeding area in the right lateral ventricle and to search for the foramen of Monro. The bottom of the third ventricle is accessed through foramen of Monro. Observing through the third ventricle's bottom, move forward to the tuber cinereum between the mammillary body and the infundibular recess as the target point. By securing the visual with the 2 mm endoscope, perform the perforation on the thin and widened area. At this time, using a pair of scissor or a forceps, small vessels are coagulated with a monopolar coagulator. After perforating, use catheter (13.5 Fr) and widen at least more than 5 mm. After expansion of the hole, check the cerebrospinal fluid's flow to each cistern. Attention is required to prevent any subdural hemorrhage caused by a rapid reduction of the ventricle size due to any excessive drainage of cerebrospinal fluid. Perform continuous saline irrigation to secure clean vision. At the last, check the ventriculostomy puncture site. Check basilar artery, short perforating arteries to the pons, superior cerebellar artery, posterior cerebral artery, pons, and others. Also, perform recheck to be sure that both the third ventricle and the arachnoid are perforated.

Complications

The complications after shunt can be classified into three types. The first is infection. The second is mechanical complication. And the last is functional complication caused by inadequate flow speed at normally operating shunt.

Shunt Infection

Nearly every prospective pediatric population shunt study has reported an infection rate of approximately 8% [8,19,20,28]. The most shunt infections appear within two months after operations. The staphylococcus epidermidis living on skin accounts for nearly two-thirds of shunt infection, and 20% is streptococcus [29]. Most of the causal organisms are found on the skin, which refers the infection after an operation is through paths of patients and medical staffs. A study by Kulkarni and associates suggested that many infections are iatrogenic, with surgical glove breaks as one of the likely and common culprits [9,21]. Especially for the ventriculoatrial shunt, bacteremia, fatal sepsis or endocarditis may occur. The principle treatment for shunt infection is to first remove the entire shunt device and perform external ventricle drainage treatment. Then, perform a new shunt procedure after complete treatment of the infection.

Mechanical Complication

Block of the shunt device is the most common mechanical complication, occurring on the proximal catheter, the valve or the distal catheter. Current series indicate that the ventricular catheter is the most common site of obstruction. Most frequently, the block will be caused by any choroid plexus or brain debris, fibrin and clotted blood sucked into the fine holes of the proximal catheter's drainage located in the ventricle. The most commonly found tissues were connective, glial, and granulomatous tissue [34]. Sometimes immediately after the operation, tissues or vein fragments in the cerebrospinal fluid may block the distal catheter. Symptoms of shunt failure include headache, vomiting, somnolence, irritability, memory changes, and the new onset or recurrence of seizure activity [11,13].

Small bowel obstruction and strangulation has been reported. Abdominal complications of ventriculoperitoneal shunt placement are common [16,32]. Perforations have occurred in nearly every viscus, and catheters have extruded from mouth, scrotum, vagina or anus [17,35].

The shunt tube is sometimes cut or moved by a separation of the connection parts of the shunt device, calcification or occurrence of chronic fatigue fracture. In one of these cases, the shunt device should be corrected with re-shunt process. Rarely, extension of the shunt tube may be required because the distal catheter becomes shorter as the patient grows.

Functional Complication

A functional complication may occur on a normally functioning shunt device depending on the drainage amount of the cerebrospinal fluid. A problem might be caused by excessive drainage of the cerebrospinal fluid due to the abdominal cavity or other causes. This is the so-called overdrainage phenomenon. This problem is related to the postural change, height and age of the patient as well as the type of valve, while it occurs frequently in old patients using low-pressure valve.

Due to excessive drainage of the cerebrospinal fluid, orthostatic hypotension with symptoms such as headache and nausea, subdural hygroma, subdural hematoma caused by bridging vein rupture or slit ventricle syndrome may occur. If postural headaches are mild, conservative managements such as hydration can often maintain the patient until the body re-equilibrates and the symptoms abate spontaneously. The subdural hygroma (< 5 mm) are usually asymptomatic and are developed to non-trauma related subdural hematoma in shunted patients by overdrainage presentation [3]. Chronic overdrainage may be induced to collapse ventricles. Slit ventricle syndrome is not symptomatic in all patients, but it may develop the mechanical obstruction of shunt. The prevalence is unknown but represents about 5% of the patients with non-normal pressure hydrocephalus. The prevalence of slit ventricle syndrome increases over time after shunt operation [1].

In children, craniosynostosis, loculation of the ventricle, seizure or intracerebral hemorrhage may occur.

Complication of the Endoscopic Third Ventriculostomy

The risk for ETV failure was ranges from 10-50% in most studies. The major complications are hemorrhage, hypothalamic injury, cerebrospinal fluid leakage, meningitis, cranial neuropathies, seizure and medical complication. Hypothalamic injuries are generally reported in studies, which include pathological weight gain and include diabetes insipidus, amenorrhea, and precocious puberty [14]. During endoscopic treatment, blood vessel damage can be the largest problem. Overall hemorrhage rate is 1%-3.6%. Just below the floor of the third ventricle, the basilar artery comes up in front of the pons. Also, on the external surface of the floor of third ventricle, important perforating arteries are located. Damaging these vessels may cause death by excessive bleeding or block the blood flow to the important parts of the pons, so that the patient may end up in a coma. If the bleeding is too much, visual security becomes hard. Unlike a craniotomy, a technical limitation for controlling of the bleeding may cause a dangerous situation. In general cases, after sufficient cleaning, the bleeding stops naturally in a while. However, even after the operation and sufficient control of the bleeding, the bleeding may happen again during the recovery process. Sometimes, if the possibility of re-bleeding is high, or the bleeding continues in small amount, the operation is completed with an external drainage tube. After observing the draining level through the tube, a following measure is performed. Damage of the brain parenchyma may occur when the endoscope is inserted. In general, almost no problem is shown. However, in a rare case, bleeding occurs on the spot the endoscope is inserted and an epileptic seizure caused by the bleeding may occur.

Long-term Complication due to Congenital Hydrocephalus

Mattihieu reported that 241 (53.7%) of 456 patients had a Karnofsky score at or above 80, meaning autonomous activity. The most common sequelaes were cognitive dysfunction in 217 (47.6%), motor weakness in 212 (46.6%), epilepsy in 105 (23.0%), behavior disturbance in 69 (15.1%), endocrine disorders in 66 (14.5%), visual loss in 62 (13.6%), pain in 35 (14.5%), and breathing problems in 12 (2.6%) cases [37]. With complications of congenital hydrocephalus, permanent brain damage may occur. Also, learning disabilities, speech problems, memory problems, short attention spans and organizational issues, visual impairments such as squint and epilepsies may occur.

REFFERENCES

[1] Bergsneider M, Miller C, Vespa PM & Hu X (2008). Surgical management of adult hydrocephalus. *Neurosurgery,* 62, 643-659

[2] Bloch O & McDermott MW (2012). Lumboperitoneal shunts for the treatment of normal pressure hydrocephalus. *J Clin Neurosci,* 19(8), 1107-1111.

[3] Boon AJ, Tans JT, Delwel EJ, Egeler-Peerdeman SM, Hanlo PW, Wurzer HA, Avezaat CJ, de Jong DA, Gooskens RH & Hermans J (1998). Dutch Normal-Pressure Hydrocephalus Study: randomized comparison of low- and medium-pressure shunts. *J Neurosurg,* 88(3), 490-495.

[4] Bret P, Guyotat J & Chazal J (2002). Is normal pressure hydrocephalus a valid concept in 2002? A reappraisal in five questions and proposal for a new designation of the syndrome as “chronic hydrocephalus.” *J Neurol Neurosurg Psychiatry,* 73(1), 9-12.

[5] Corkill RG & Cadoux-Hudson TA (1999). Normal pressure hydrocephalus: developments in determining surgical prognosis. *Curr Opin Neurol*, 12(6), 671-677.

[6] Czosnyka M, Czosnyka ZH, Whitfield PC, Donovan T & Pickard JD (2001). Age dependence of cerebrospinal pressure-volume compensation in patients with hydrocephalus. *J Neurosurg,* 94(3), 482-486

[7] Di Rocco C, Massimi L & Tamburrini G (2006). Shunts vs. endoscopic third ventriculostomy in infants: are there different types and/or complications? A review. *Childs Nerv Syst,* 22(12), 1573-1589.

[8] Drake JM, Kestle JR, Milner R, Cinalli G, Boop F, Piatt J Jr, Haines S, Schiff SJ, Cochrane DD, Steinbok P & MacNeil N (1998). Randomized trial of cerebrospinal fluid shunt valve design in pediatric hydrocephalus. *Neurosurgery,* 43(2), 294-303.

[9] Drake JM (2006). Does double gloving prevent cerebrospinal fluid shunt infection. *J Neurosurg,* 104(1 Suppl), 3-4.

[10] Drake JM, Kulkarni AV & Kestle J (2009). Endoscopic third ventriculostomy versus ventriculoperitoneal shunt in pediatric patients: a decision analysis. *Childs Nerv Syst,* 25(4), 467-472

[11] Faillace WJ & Canady AI (1990). Cerebrospinal fluid shunt malfunction signaled by new or recurrent seizures. *Childs Nerv Syst,* 6(1), 37-40.

[12] Gilmore H. Medical treatment of hydrocephalus. In: Editor Scott RM, *Hydrocephalus.* Baltimore: Williams and Wilkins; 1990; 37-46

[13] Hack CH, Enrile BG, Donat JF & Kosnik E (1990). Seizures in relation to shunt dysfunction in children with meningomyelocele. *J Pediatr,* 116(1), 57-60.

[14] Hader WJ, Walker RL, Myles ST & Hamilton M (2008). Complications of endoscopic third ventriculostomy in previously shunted patients. *Neurosurgery,* 63(1 Suppl), 168-174

[15] Hakim S & Adams RD (1965). The special clinical problem of symptomatic hydrocephalus with normal cerebrospinal fluid pressure. Observations on cerebrospinal fluid hydrodynamics. *J Neurol Sci,* 2(4), 307-327.

[16] Hlavin ML, Mapstone TB & Gauderer MW (1990). Small bowel obstruction secondary to incomplete removal of a ventriculoperitoneal shunt: Case report. *Neurosurgery,* 26(3), 526-528.

[17] Hornig GW & Shillito J Jr. (1990). Intestinal perforation by peritoneal shunt tubing: Report of two cases. *Surg Neurol,* 33(4), 288-290.

[18] Ignelzi RJ & Kirsch WM (1975). Follow-up analysis of ventriculoperitoneal and ventricuoatrial shunts for hydrocephalus. *J Neurosurg,* 42(6), 679-682.

[19] Kestle JR, Drake JM, Cochrane DD, Milner R, Walker ML, Abbott R 3rd & Boop FA (2003). Endoscopic Shunt Insertion Trial participants: Lack of benefit of endoscopic ventriculoperitoneal shunt insertion: a multicenter randomized trial. *J Neurosurg,* 98(2), 284-290.

[20] Kestle JR & Walker ML (2005). A multicenter prospective cohort study of the Strata valve for the management of hydrocephalus in pediatric patients. *J Neurosurg,* 102(2 Suppl),141-145.

[21] Kulkarni AV, Drake JM & Lamberti-Pasculli M (2001). Cerebrospinal fluid shunt infection: a prospective study of risk factors. *J Neurosurg,* 94(2),195-201.

[22] Kulkarni AV, Drake JM, Mallucci CL, Sgouros S, Roth J, Constantini S & Canadian Pediatric Neurosurgery Study Group (2009). Endoscopic third ventriculostomy in the treatment of childhood hydrocephalus. *J Pediatr,* 155(2), 254-259.

[23] Lifshutz JI & Johnson WD (2001). History of hydrocephalus and its treatments. *Neurosurg Focus,* 11(2), E1.

[24] Momjian S, Owler BK, Czosnyka Z, Czosnyka M, Pena A & Pickard JD (2004). Pattern of white matter regional cerebral blood flow and autoregulation in normal pressure hydrocephalus. *Brain,*127(5), 965-972.

[25] O'Brien DF, Javadpour M, Collins DR, Spennato P & Mallucci CL (2005). Endoscopic third ventriculostomy: an outcome analysis of primary cases and procedures performed after ventriculoperitoneal shunt malfunction. *J Neurosurg,* 103 (5 Suppl), 393-400.

[26] Oertel JM, Baldauf J, Schroeder HW & Gaab MR (2009). Endoscopic options in children: experience with 134 procedures. *J Neurosurg Pediatr,* 3(2), 81-89.

[27] Schmitt PJ & Jane JA Jr.(2012). A lesson in history: the evolution of endoscopic third Ventriculostomy. *Neurosurg Focus,* 33(2), E11.

[28] Pollack IF, Albright AL & Adelson PD (1999). A randomized, controlled study of a programmable shunt valve versus a conventional valve for patients with hydrocephalus. Hakim-Medos Investigator Group. *Neurosurgery,* 45(6), 1399-1408.

[29] Quigley MR, Reigel DH & Kortyna R (1989). Cerebrospinal fluid shunt infections. Report of 41 cases and a critical review of the literature. *Pediatr Neurosci,* 15(3), 111-120.

[30] Ray P, Jallo GI, Kim RY, Kim BS, Wilson S, Kothbauer K & Abbott R (2005). Endoscopic third ventriculostomy for tumor related hydrocephalus in pediatric population. *Neurosurg Focus,* 15;19(6), E8.

[31] Relkin N, Marmarou A, Klinge P, Bergsneider M & Black PM (2005). Diagnosing idiopathic normal-pressure hydrocephalus. *Neurosurgery,* 57(3 Suppl), S4-16.

[32] Scott RM. Preventing and treating shunt complications. In: Editor Scott Rm. Hydrocephalus. *Baltimore: Williams and Wikins;* 1990; 115-121.

[33] Silverberg GD (2004). Normal pressure hydrocephalus (NPH): ischaemia, CSF stagnation or both. *Brain,* 127(5), 947-948.

[34] Sekhar LM, Moossy J & Guthkelch AN (1982). Malfunctioning ventriculoperitoneal shunts: Clinical and pathological features. *J Neurosurg,* 56(3), 411-416.

[35] Touho H, Nakauchi M, Tasawa T, Nakagawa J & Karasawa J (1987). Intrahepatic migration of a peritoneal shunt catheter: case report. *Neurosurgery,* 21(2), 258-259.

[36] Weller RO & Shulman K (1972). Infantile hydrocephalus: clinical, histological, and ultrastructural study of brain damage. *J Neurosurg,* 36(3), 255-265.

[37] Vinchon M, Baroncini M & Delestret I (2012). Adult outcome of pediatric hydrocephalus. *Childs Nerv Syst,* 28(6), 847-854.

[38] Volpe J. *Neurology of the Newborn,* ed 2. Philadelphia: WB Saunders; 1987.

In: Hydrocephalus
Editor: Amaya Velazquez

ISBN: 978-1-62100-453-0

Chapter 3

NORMAL-PRESSURE HYDROCEPHALUS: A COMMON SOURCE OF ELDERLY INCONTINENCE WITH BRAIN ETIOLOGY

Ryuji Sakakibara,[1*] Fuyuki Tateno,[1] Masahiko Kishi,[1] Yohei Tsuyusaki,[1] Tomoyuki Uchiyama,[2] Tomonori Yamanishi[2] and Tatsuya Yamamoto[3]

[1]Neurology, Internal Medicine, Sakura Medical Center, Toho University, Sakura, Japan

[2]Continence Center, Dokkyo Medical College, Tochigi, Japan

[3]Neurology, Chiba University, Chiba, Japan

ABSTRACT

This paper reviewed a common source of elderly incontinence with brain etiology, normal-pressure hydrocephalus (NPH), from auro-neurological point of view. This disease manifests with gait disturbance, dementia, and urinary incontinence as a clinical triad. Urinary frequency/ urgency (overactive bladder) often precedes urinary incontinence in this disease, and in some patients may be the early manifestation. While NPHis less common than white matter disease in the elderly, at

---

* Corresponding author: Ryuji Sakakibara, MD, PhD, Associate Professor, Neurology, Internal Medicine, Sakura Medical Center, Toho University, 564-1 Shimoshizu, Sakura, 285-8741 Japan. Telephone: +81-43-462-8811 ext. 2323 Fax: +81-43-487-4246, E-mail: sakakibara@ sakura.med.toho-u.ac.jp.

approximately one-tenth the prevalence, it is particularly important because the symptoms can be reversed by shunt surgery or endoscopic third ventriculostomy. Bladder overactivity due to frontal hypofunction, which normally tonically inhibits the micturition reflex, commonly underlies OAB in this disease. Recent brain SPECT imaging has shown close relationship between frontal hypofunction and OAB, both of which are dynamically improved after shunt surgery in this disease.

Keywords: Normal-pressure hydrocephalus, geriatric incontinence, overactive bladder, shunt surgery, anticholinergic drug

INTRODUCTION

Urinary incontinence is a major concern in geriatric populations, which have grown rapidly in recent decades. In addition, the incidence of urinary frequency/urgency (also called overactive bladder, OAB), with or without incontinence, in the general population over 40 years in age is common [1,2,3], and increases significantly with age. It is widely acknowledged that urinary frequency and poor bladder control has an impact on quality of life [4] and that bladder dysfunction in elderly persons adds to their caretakers' burdens and is an important factor leading to institutionalization [4]. The mechanisms of OAB and urinary incontinence in the frail elderly are multifactorial, and may include age-related changes in the bladder itself [4], or central nervous system changes in nervating the bladder [5]. Normal-pressure hydrocephalus (NPH) is a relatively common brain disease in the elderly that can be treated by shunt surgery or endoscopic third ventriculostomy [6,7]. This disease was first described by Hakim and Adams in 1965 [6,7].

Since then, the clinical triad of gait disturbance, dementia, and OAB/ urinary incontinence in NPH is widely recognized, and is a common source of elderly incontinence with brain etiology. This paper reviews NPH from auro-neurological point of view.

BLADDER DYSFUNCTION IN NPH

NPH is characterized by a clinical presentation of gait disturbance, dementia, and OAB/ urinary incontinence, combined with dilated cerebral ventricles and normal cerebrospinal fluid (CSF) pressure [8]. Studies analyzingthe intracranial hydrodynamics related to the pulse pressure, etc. [9], have indicated that CSF pressure in NPH is not truly "normal", although there is an expected low threshold range. The clinical triad of this disorder is very much akin to those of cerebral white matter disease (WMD).

Therefore, before performing brain imaging, we have to think about NPH as well as cerebral WMD. Since the first description of NPH [6,7], the effectiveness of the diversion of CSF flow by shunt operation in treating this syndrome is well documented [8,10].

Recent population-based magnetic resonance imaging (MRI) studies also suggest that the incidence of NPH, or asymptomatic ventriculomegaly with feature so fidiopathic NPH on MRI (AVIM), to be around 1% (0.51– 2.9%) in the general population of persons over 65 years of age [11,12].

We recently studied the bladder function in 42 idiopathic NPH (iNPH) patients [13]. They were diagnosed to have iNPHby clinical symptoms/signs (gait, cognitive, and urinary disorders) with typical imaging features (ventricular enlargement) and normal cerebrospinal fluid pressureby a spinal tap test (normal range of the opening pressure, 90– 180 mmH_2O [14]). The subjects included 36 men and 6 women; mean age, 72 years (62– 83 years). As a result, lower urinary tract symptoms (LUTS) were seen in 93% of patients; these symptoms included storage symptoms in 93% of patients (nocturnal urinary frequency, 64%; urinary urgency (OAB), 64%; urgency urinary incontinence, 57%; diurnal urinary frequency, 36%) and voiding symptoms in 71% (retardation in initiating urination, 50%; prolongation/poor flow, 50%; sensation of post-void residual (PVR), 29%; straining, 21%; and intermittency, 14%) (Table 1).

As shown above, the majority of our patients (93%) had storage symptoms, and some had OAB without urinary incontinence. These findings indicate that urinary urgency/frequency might precede urinary incontinence in iNPH.

Therefore, for both urologists and non-urological clinicians, it is important to think about NPH when we see elderly patients with OAB. Among the clinical triad of NPH, urinary incontinence has been reported to be present in 68% (103/151), which is less common than either gait, in 91% (138/151), or dementia, in 86% (130/151) [8], and is regarded a late symptom [15].

However, as in cases of cerebral WMD, not urinary incontinence but gait disturbance and OAB might be the early manifestations of NPH.

Table 1. Urodynamic findings of normal-pressure hydrocephalus

total number of patients		42	
		average	range
free flow			
voided volume		102.5	19-250
maximum flow	(ml/s)	11.7	3-33
post-void residual	(ml)	42.1	0-228
post-void residual>100 ml		14.3%	female 3 (105-228 ml); male 3 (100-180 ml)
cystometry			
first sensation	(ml)	134.1	0-300
bladder capacity	(ml)	200.8	20-470
detrusor overactivity		95.2%	

Cited from ref. 13.

Cause of Bladder Dysfunction in NPH

We also performed urodynamics in 42 iNPH patients [13] (Table 1). In the voiding phase, free flowmetry revealed that the maximum flow rate (Qmax) was low (<10 cm/s) in 40% of patients and normal (>10 cm/s) in 60%, and the mean Qmax was 11.7 ml/s. Measurement of post-void residual (PVR)by trans urethral catheterization revealed that PVR volume was elevated (>30 ml) in 43% of patients and normal (< 30 ml) in 57%, and the mean PVR volume was 42.1 ml.

Among patients whose PVR was increased, PVR >100 ml was noted in 6 patients (3 women [105-228 ml], 3 men [100-180 ml]). In the storage phase, bladder volume at the first sensation was low (< 100 ml) in 33% of patients, normal (100-300 ml) in 67%, high (> 300 ml) in none, and the mean bladder volume at the first sensation was 134 ml. In contrast, bladder capacity was decreased (< 200 ml) in 57%, normal (200–600 ml) in 43%, and increased (> 600 ml) in none, and the mean bladder capacity was 200 ml. DO was seen in 95% of patients.

Therefore, the significant urodynamic abnormality that underlies bladder dysfunction in iNPH appears to be DO, which was noted in 95.2% of our 42 patients. Previous reports of NPH have indicated results similar to our own, although the number of cases included in these reports has been small (range, 4-12 cases) [16,17]. The reported frequency of DO has ranged from 63% to 100% [16,17].

Although DO is not uncommon in general older populations [18,19], the high prevalence of DO in NPH cases strongly suggests altered brain autonomic control in this disorder.

Cerebral Control of the Bladder and How It Is Affected by NPH

DO in NPH patients reflects a loss of inhibition of the micturition reflex, suggesting a primary brain autonomic dysfunction [20]. Recent functional neuroimaging in normal volunteers has shown that the anterior cingulate, prefrontal cortex and insula are activated in response to bladder filling as compared with an empty bladder. [22,23,24] Although NPH is a diffuse brain disease with dilated ventricles, hypoperfusion in the frontal lobe has been documented in NPH patients using PET [24,25], single-photon emission computed tomography (SPECT) [26], and perfusion-weighted MRI [27]. Therefore, it is possible that the frontal lobe is the anatomical substrate for the development of urinary incontinence in NPH. We recently studied the correlation between urinary incontinence and frontal lobe function in iNPH by SPECT and statistical brain mapping [28]. Urinary symptoms were observed and [^{123}I]-iodoamphetamine (IMP)-SPECT imaging was performed in 97 patients with clinico-radiologically definite iNPH. The patients included 56 men and 41 women; mean age, 74 years. The study calculated and visualized the statistical difference in normalized mean tracer counts between patients with urinary dysfunction of severer degrees (≥grade 2/4) and milder degrees (≤grade 1/4) according to the urinary subscales of the iNPH grading scales [13,28]. As a result, there was a significant decrease in tracer activity in the right-side-dominant bilateral frontal cortex and the left inferior temporal gyrus in the severe urinary dysfunction group ($p<0.05$) (Figure 1 upper row). In order to minimize the effects of gait and cognitive dysfunction, we performed a similar analysis among subjects with little or no such dysfunction, and obtained the same results ($p<0.05$) as described above. As shown above, there is a link between right frontal hypoperfusion and urinary dysfunction in iNPH. In addition, right frontal hypoperfusion related with urinary dysfunction was observed in the subgroup of patients with adjusted gait or cognitive grades. The facts indicate that urinary dysfunction might occur independently of gait or cognitive disturbance in iNPH.

In addition, there was also a significant increase in tracer activity in the bilateral posterior cingulate gyrus, left pontine-mesencephalic area, etc., related with urinary dysfunction in iNPH ($p<0.05$) (Figure 1 lower row). Recent functional PET in Parkinson's disease with DO [29] and fMRI in idiopathic DO [30] showed that cortical activation with DO was decreased in the frontal pole and the prefrontal cortex; whereas it was higher than in normal volunteers in the supplementary motor area (SMA), which is close to the medial frontal and parietal gyrus as we have shown herein. The SMA activation associated with DO might reflect simultaneous pelvic floor contraction against the DO in order to maintain urinary continence. [29]

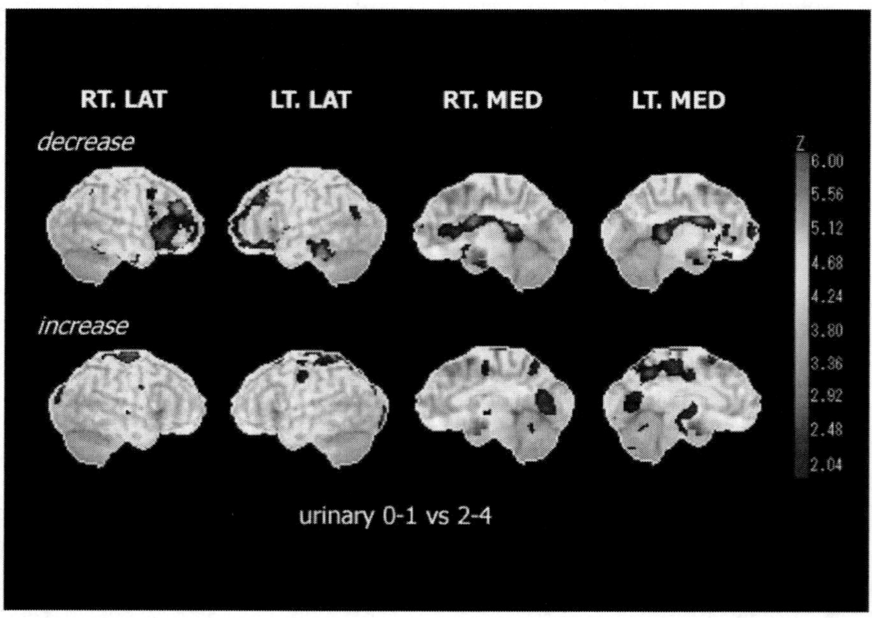

Cited from ref. 28.

Figure 1. 3D-SSP maps of differences of cerebral blood flow as measured by [123I]-labeled IMP in NPH patients with urinary grades of 0-1 and 2-4 (n=97).
Upper row: decrease of tracer accumulation in the group with severe urinary dysfunction as compared to mild urinary dysfunction; lower row: increase of tracer accumulation in the group with severe urinary dysfunction. Colored areas indicate the areas of statistically significant difference ($p<0.05$).

SHUNT SURGERY OF NPH ON BLADDER FUNCTION

Importantly, bladder dysfunction and frontal lobe hypoperfusion in NPH can be reversed after shunt surgery. The recovery rate of OAB and urinary incontinence in iNPH ranges around 20-80%. Among them, cerebral perfusion in the prefrontal cortex and mid-cingulate gyrus tended to return to normal, particularly in patients with good OAB/incontinence recovery (data not shown).

Nowadays, endoscopic third ventriculostomy (ETV) is being increasingly acknowledged as an alternative treatment for ventriculoperitoneal/lumbar peritoneal shunt, or even as a first-line treatment, in selected patients [31].

SYMPTOMATIC TREATMENT OF OAB AND URINARY INCONTINENCE OF BRAIN ETIOLOGIES

Urological causes are an important cause for incontinence in the elderly. DO may occur in men with benign prostatic enlargement; however, in 25-93% of prostatectomy cases, detrusor overactivity is reported to remain unchanged after surgery, the figures increase with age [30,32]. Concomitant cerebral ischemic white matter disease (WMD, also referred to as 'vascular incontinence') [33] are reported in this group [34] and are likely to contribute to DO. Elderly women may present with stress incontinence, which can be differentiated by history.

There are no established regimens to treat OAB in NPH, particularly in patients who have not undergone shunt surgery or those who did not respond well to shunt surgery. Medications used to treat elderly OAB and urinary incontinence of brain etiologiesinclude anticholinergic agents such as oxybutynin, propiverine, detrusitol, solifenacin, and imidafenacin [1,35]. Mori et al. [36] performed urodynamics in 46 dementia patients, and found DO in 91% of patients with WMD and 58% of Alzheimer's disease patients. They conducted an open trial with 20 mg/day of propiverine hydrochloride for 2 weeks irrespective of the presence of DO, and found increased bladder capacity or lessened frequency of incontinence in 40% of patients. Both groups responded almost equally, and patients with DO showed a more satisfactory response. Treatment for urinary frequency/urgency may be particularly of benefit in subjects without marked immobility or dementia.

The use of medications with anticholinergic side-effects in the elderly is of concern, particularly when there is a risk of exacerbating cognitive impairment. Crossing the blood-brain barrier (BBB), they can act at the M1-muscarinic receptors in the cerebral cortex and hippocampus, or M4-receptors in the basal ganglia. Factors predisposing patients to cognitive side effects include 1) central muscarinic receptor affinity, e.g., high M1-receptor selectivity; and 2) permeability across the BBB: size, lipid solubility, fewer hydrogen bonds, neutral or low degree of ionization and a small number of rotatable bonds [37,38]. Darifenacin is an M3-selective antagonist and thus has less marked cognitive side effects while trospium, a quaternary amine, has high polarity and therefore poor permeability across the BBB [39,40,41]. Other common anticholinergic side-effects are dryness of the mouth (M3) and constipation (M2,3). Extended-release formulations may lessen these adverse effects [42,43]. It has been recently shown that the addition of propiverineto donepezil ameliorated OAB without worsening cognitive function in elderly OAB patients with dementia [44]. Mirabeglon, a novel adrenergic beta-3 receptor agonist, seems to be promising for lessening DO with fewer central side effects [45].

Conclusion

This paper reviewed NPH, a common source of elderly incontinence with brain etiology, from auro- neurological point of view. This disease manifests with gait disturbance, dementia, and urinary incontinence as a clinical triad. OAB often precedes urinary incontinence in this disease, and in some patients may be the early manifestation. While NPH is less common than WMD (also referred to as 'vascular incontinence'), at approximately one-tenth the prevalence, it is particularly important because the symptoms can be reversed by shunt surgery or endoscopic third ventriculostomy. Bladder overactivity due to frontal hypofunction, which normally tonically inhibits the micturition reflex, commonly underlies OAB in this disease. Recent brain SPECT imaging has shown close relationship between frontal hypofunction and OAB, both of which are dynamically improved after shunt surgery in this disease.

References

[1] Milsom, I., Abrams, P., Cardozo, L., Roberts, R. G., Thuèroff, J., Wein, A. J. How widespread are the symptoms of an overactive bladder and how are they managed? A population-based prevalence study. *BJU International* 2001; 87: 760-766.

[2] Stewart, W. F., Van Rooyen, J. B., Cundiff, G. W., Abrams, P., Herzog, A. R., Corey, R., Hunt, T. L., Wein, A. J. Prevalence and burden of

overactive bladder in the United States. *World J. Urol.* 2003; 20: 327-336.

[3] Homma, Y., Yamaguchi, O., Hayashi, K., the Members of the Neurogenic Bladder Society Committee. An epidemiological survey of overactive bladder symptoms in Japan. *BJU International* 2005; 96: 1314-1318.

[4] Irwin, D. E., Milsom, I., Kopp, Z., Abrams, P., Cardozo, L. Impact of overactive bladder symptoms on employment, social interactions and emotional well-being in six European countries. *BJU International* 2005; 97: 96-100.

[5] Resnick, N. M. Urinary incontinence. *Lancet.* 1995 346: 94-99.

[6] Hakim, S., Adams, R. D. The special clinical problem of symptomatic occult hydrocephalus with normal cerebrospinal pressure. *J. Neurol. Sci.* 1965; 2: 307-327.

[7] Adams, R. D., Fisher, C. M., Hakim, S., Ojeman, R. G., Sweet, W. H. Symptomatic occult hydrocephalus with 'normal' cerebrospinal pressure. *N Eng. J. Med.* 1965; 273: 117-126.

[8] Marmarou, A., Black, P., Bergsneider, M., Klinge, P., Relkin, N.; International NPH Consultant Group. International NPH Consultant Group. Guidelines for management of idiopathic normal pressure hydrocephalus: progress to date. *Acta Neurochir. Suppl.* 2005; 95: 237-240.

[9] Greitz, D. Radiological assessment of hydrocephalus: new theories and implications for therapy. *Neurosurg. Rev.* 2004; 27: 145–165.

[10] Ishii, K., Hashimoto, M., Hayashida, K., Hashikawa, K., Chang, C. C., Nakagawara, J., Nakayama, T., Mori, S., Sakakibara, R. A multicenter brain perfusion SPECT study evaluating idiopathic normal-pressure hydrocephalus on neurological improvement. *Dementia and Geriatric Cognitive Disorders* 2011;32:1-10.

[11] Hiraoka, K., Meguro, K., Mori, E. Prevalence of idiopathic normal-pressure hydrocephalus in the elderly population of a Japanese rural community. *Neurol. Med. Chir.* (Tokyo). 2008; 48: 197-199.

[12] Iseki, C., Kawanami, T., Nagasawa, H., Wada, M., Koyama, S., Kikuchi, K., Arawaka, S., Kurita, K., Daimon, M., Mori, E., Kato, T. Asymptomatic ventriculomegaly with features of idiopathic normal pressure hydrocephalus on MRI (AVIM) in the elderly: a prospective study in a Japanese population. *J. Neurol. Sci.* 2009;277:54-57.

[13] Sakakibara, R., Kanda, T., Sekido, T., Uchiyama, T., Awa, Y., Ito, T., Liu, Z., Yamamoto, T., Yamanishi, T., Yuasa, T., Shirai, K., Hattori, T.

Mechanism of bladder dysfunction in idiopathic normal pressure hydrocephalus. *Neurourol. Urodyn.* 2008; 27: 507-510.

[14] Yuh, E. L., Dillon, W. P. Intracranial hypotension and intracranial hypertension. *Neuroimaging Clin. N Am.* 2010; 20:597-617.

[15] Meier, U., Zeilinger, F. S., Kintzel, D. Signs, symptoms and course of normal pressure hydrocephalus in comparison with cerebral atrophy. *Acta Neurochir.* (Wien) 1999; 141: 1039-1048.

[16] Jonas, S., Brown, J. Neurogenic bladder in normal pressure hydrocephalus. *Urology* 1975; 5: 44-50.

[17] Ahlberg, J., Noren, L., Blomstrand, C., Wikkelso, C. Outcome of shunt operation on urinary incontinence in normal pressure hydrocephalus predicted by lumber puncture. *J. Neurol. Neurosurg. Psychiatry* 1988; 51: 105-108.

[18] Malone-Lee, J. G., Wahedna, I. Characterisation of detrusor contractile function in relation to old age. *Br. J. Urol.* 1993; 72: 873-880.

[19] Resnick, N. M., Elbadawi, A., Yalla, S. V. Age and the lower urinary tract: what is normal? *Neurourol. Urodyn.* 1995; 14: 577-579.

[20] De Groat, W. C. Integrative control of the lower urinary tract: preclinical perspective. *Br. J. Pharmacol.* 2006; 147: S25–S40.

[21] DasGupta, R., Kavia, R. B., Fowler, C. J. Cerebral mechanisms and voiding function. *BJU Int.* 2007; 99: 731-734.

[22] Sakakibara, R., Tsunoyama, K., Takahashi, O., Sugiyama, M., Kishi, M., Ogawa, E., Uchiyama, T., Yamamoto, T., Yamanishi, T., Awa, Y., Yamaguchi, C. Real-time measurement of oxyhemoglobin concentration changes in the frontal micturition area: an fNIRS study. *Neurourol. Urodyn.* 2010; 29: 757-764.

[23] Fowler, C. J., Griffiths, D. J. A decade of functional brain imaging applied to bladder control. *Neurourol. Urodyn.* 2010; 29: 49-55.

[24] Momjian, S., Owler, B. K., Czosnyka, Z., Czosnyka, M., Pena, A., Pickard, J. D. Pattern of white matter regional cerebral blood flow and autoregulation in normal pressure hydrocephalus. *Brain* 2004; 127: 965-972.

[25] Owler, B. K., Momjian, S., Czosnyka, Z., Czosnyka, M., Pena, A., Harris, N. G., Smielewski, P., Fryer, T., Donovan, T., Coles, J., Carpenter, A., Pickard, J. D. Normal pressure hydrocephalus and cerebral blood flow: a PET study of baseline values. *J. Cereb. Blood Flow Metab.* 2004; 24: 17-23.

[26] Sasaki, H., Ishii, K., Kono, A., Miyamoto, N., Fukuda, T., Shimada, K., Ohkawa, S., Kawaguchi, T., Mori, E. Cerebral perfusion pattern of

idiopathic normal pressure hydrocephalus studied by SPECT and statistical brain mapping. *Ann. Nucl. Med.* 2007; 21: 39-45.

[27] Walter, C., Hertel, F., Neumann, E., Morsdorf, M. Alteration of cerebral perfusion in patients with idiopathic normal pressure hydrocephalus measured by 3D perfusion weighted magnetic resonance imaging. *J. Neurol.* 2005; 252: 1465-1471.

[28] Sakakibara, R., Uchida, Y., Ishii, K., Kazui, H., Hashimoto, M., Ishikawa, M., Yuasa, T., Kishi, M., Ogawa, E., Tateno, F., Uchiyama, T., Yamamoto, T., Yamanishi, T., Terada, H.; the members of SINPHONI (Study of Idiopathic Normal Pressure Hydrocephalus On Neurological Improvement). Correlation of right frontal hypoperfusion and urinary dysfunction in iNPH: A SPECT study. *Neurourol. Urodyn.* 2011 Oct. 28. [Epub. ahead of print]

[29] Kitta, T., Kakizaki, H., Furuno, T., Moriya, K., Tanaka, H., Shiga, T., Tamaki, N., Yabe, I., Sasaki, H., Nonomura, K. Brain activation during detrusor overactivity in patients with Parkinson's disease: a positron emission tomography study. *J. Urol.* 2006; 175: 994-998.

[30] Griffiths, D., Derbyshire, S., Stenger, A., Resnick, N. Brain control of normal and overactive bladder. *J. Urol.* 2005; 174: 1862-1867.

[31] Rangel-Castilla, L., Barber, S., Zhang, Y. J. The role of endoscopic third ventriculostomy in the treatment of communicating hydrocephalus. *World Neurosurg.* 2011 Nov. 7. [Epub. ahead of print]

[32] Gormley, E. A., Griffiths, D. J., McCracken, P. N., Harrison, G. M., McPhee, M. S. Effect of transurethral resection of the prostate on detrusor instability and urge incontinence in elderly males. *Neurourol. Urodyn.* 1993; 12: 445–453.

[33] Sakakibara, R., Panicker, J., Fowler, C. J., Tateno, F., Kishi, M., Tsuyusaki, Y., Ogawa, E., Uchiyama, T., Yamamoto, T. Vascular incontinence: incontinence in the elderly due to ischemic white matter changes. *Neurology International* 2012: in press.

[34] Sakakibara, R., Hamano, S., Uchiyama, T., Liu, Z., Yamanishi, T., Hattori, T. Do BPH patients have neurogenic detrusor dysfunction? A uro-neurological assessment. *Urol. Int.* 2005; 74: 44-50.

[35] Homma, Y., Yamaguchi, O., for the Imidafenacin Study Group. A randomized, double-blind, placebo- and propiverine-controlled trial of the novel antimuscarinic agent imidafenacin in Japanese patients with overactive bladder. *Int. J. Urol.* 2009; 16: 499–506.

[36] Mori, S., Kojima, M., Sakai, Y., Nakajima, K. Bladder dysfunction in dementia patients showing urinary incontinence; evaluation with

cystometry and treatment with propiverine hydrochloride. *Jpn. J. Geriat.* 1999; 36:489–494.

[37] Wardlaw, J. M. Blood-brain barrier and cerebral small vessel disease. *J. Neurol. Sci.* 2010; 299: 66-71.

[38] Scheife, R., Takeda, M. Central nervous system safety of anticholinergic drugs for the treatment of overactive bladder in the elderly. *Clin. Ther.* 2005; 27: 144-153.

[39] Wagg, C., Verdejo, U., Molander, U. Review of cognitive impairment with antimuscarinicagents in elderly patients with overactive bladder. *Int. J. Clin. Pract.*, 2010; 64: 1279–1286.

[40] Pagoria, D., O'Connor, R. C., Guralnick, M. L. Antimuscarinic drugs: review of the cognitive impact when used to treat overactive bladder in elderly patients. *Curr. Urol. Rep.* 2011; 12:351–357.

[41] Chancellor, M., Boone, T. Anticholinergics foroveractive bladder therapy: central nervous system effects. *CNS Neurosci. Ther.* 2012;18:167-174.

[42] Sakakibara, R., Uchiyama, T., Yamanishi, T., Kishi, M. Dementia and lower urinary dysfunction: with a reference to anticholinergic use in elderly population. *Int. J. Urol.* 2008; 15: 778-788.

[43] Chu, F. M., Dmochowski, R. R., Lama, D. J., Anderson, R. U., Sand, P. K. Extended-release formulations of oxybutynin and tolterodine exhibit similar central nervous system tolerability profiles: A subanalysis of data from the OPERA trial. *Am. J. Obstet. Gynecol.* 2005; 192: 1849-1855.

[44] Sakakibara, R., Ogata, T., Uchiyama, T., Kishi, M., Ogawa, E., Isaka, S., Yuasa, J., Yamamoto, T., Ito, T., Yamanishi, T., Awa, Y., Yamaguchi, C., Takahashi, O. How to manage overactive bladder in elderly individuals with dementia? A combined use of donepezil, a central AChE inhibitor, and propiverine, a peripheral muscarine receptor antagonist. *J. Am. Geriatr. Soc.* 2009;57:1515-1517.

[45] Tyagi, P., Tyagi, V., Chancellor, M. Mirabegron: a safety review. *Expert Opin. Drug Saf.* 2011;10:287-294.

In: Hydrocephalus
Editor: Amaya Velazquez
ISBN: 978-1-62100-453-0

Chapter 4

PEDIATRIC HYDROCEPHALUS

Wen-Shan Sung*, Aden McLaughlin and Sharon Gabizon
Department of Neurosurgery, Gold Coast Hospital, Queensland, Australia

ABSTRACT

Hydrocephalus can occur in infancy and it often coexists with many congenital and acquired brain disorders. The diagnosis and management of hydrocephalus present common problems in pediatric patients. Diagnosis of pediatric hydrocephalus often require high index of suspension and early detection with institution of treatment can prove to be pivotal in order to prevent long-term complication. Surgery still remains as mainstream treatment for pediatric hydrocephalus. Various surgical approaches have been advocated, and VP shunt is by far the most commonly practiced procedure worldwide. Patients with implanted VP shunts may present with complex and challenging problems that include infection and obstruction of the shunt.

Therefore insertion of a VP shunt represents a lifetime commitment for the child and family and the decision to treat can be difficult and it should not be taken lightly. Mortality has significantly reduced with modern surgical technique, yet there is still much long-term morbidity associated with the disorder. Multidisciplinary planning and close follow-

* Corresponding Author: Wen-Shan Sung. Address: Department of Neurosurgery, Gold Coast Hospital, 108 Nerang Street, Southport, Queensland, 4215, Australia; Phone: 61-0401487846, Email: wssung@gmail.com.

up is needed to ensure the maximal developmental potential of these children.

In this chapter we will discuss the clinical features, diagnosis, and management of pediatric hydrocephalus.

INTRODUCTION

Hydrocephalus is the pathologic enlargement of the cerebral ventricles caused by a mismatch between the production of cerebrospinal fluid (CSF) and its absorption.

Classically, hydrocephalus has been divided into two subtypes: communicating and non-communicating. Non-communicating hydrocephalus results from obstruction of CSF within the ventricular system, whereas communicating hydrocephalus implies that there is free-flowing CSF within the ventricular system but absorption at the subarachnoid villi and granulations is impaired. Hydrocephalus may cause pathological changes to brain morphology, microstructure, circulation, biochemistry, metabolism, and maturation [1].

Although treatment does not always reverse the damage, untreated hydrocephalus will lead to progressive neurological decline and eventually death. In essence, once the diagnosis is confirmed a definitive treatment should not be delayed.

ETIOLOGY

Hydrocephalus can affect all ages, from infants to elderly people. In pediatric patients, hydrocephalus may present at birth and it may be caused by either environmental influence during fetal development or genetic predisposition. Acquired hydrocephalus develops at the time of birth or at some point afterward. This type of hydrocephalus can affect individuals of all ages and is usually caused by injury or disease. Table 1 shows the common causes of congenital and acquired pediatric hydrocephalus.

Congenital hydrocephalus has an estimated incidence of about 3 to 4 per 1000 live births [2]. The most common causes of congenital hydrocephalus are due to structural defects such as Chiari malformations and aqueductal stenosis [3]. Dandy Walker malformation is less common but also an important cause of infantile hydrocephalus.

Table 1. Common Causes of Pediatric Hydrocephalus

Congenital • Chiari malformation • Aqueductal stenosis (X linked) • Dandy-Walker complex • Congenital arachnoid cysts
Acquired • Intraventricular Haemorrhage • Infection • Traumatic head injury • Tumour

The Dandy-Walker malformation is a cystic dilatation of the fourth ventricle following partial or complete agenesis of the cerebellar vermis, which leads to obstruction of CSF outflow though atresia of foramina of the fourth ventricle. It is not uncommon that some midline and posterior fossa arachnoid cysts in newborn may also cause obstructive hydrocephalus. These congenital arachnoid cysts are commonly found in suprasellar area, quadrigeminal cistern, or cerebellopontine angle. Additionally, intrauterine infections, especially toxoplasmosis, rubella, cytomegalovirus, and syphilis, may be associated with congenital hydrocephalus as a consequence of aqueduct gliosis.

Intraventricular hemorrhage (IVH) in premature newborn is common and is related to the degree of prematurity and the birth weight [4]. IVH is the result of vascular instability of cerebral vessels in the germinal matrix at the level of the head of the caudate in the premature infant. Bleeding of these vessels may extend into ventricles with subsequent ventricular dilatation. After the newborn period, common causes of hydrocephalus are hemorrhage, and post-viral or post-bacterial meningitis.

The mechanism of formation of hydrocephalus secondary to hemorrhage in other age groups is the same as for premature infants described above, except that the origin of bleeding is different and may be due to rupture of an AV malformation, or as a result of a traumatic injury. In bacterial or viral meningitis, impaired CSF absorption at arachnoid granulations by cellular debris or its subsequent scaring of meninges may also produce non-communicating hydrocephalus. Furthermore, the tendency for children's brain tumor to occur in the posterior fossa and midline leads to a high incidence of associated hydrocephalus.

CLINICAL FEATURES

Clinical features of hydrocephalus vary with age, disease progression, and individual's tolerance to excessive CSF. Table 2 summarizes a list of signs and symptoms of hydrocephalus in different age group.

In infants before 2 years of age, hydrocephalus will invariably present with rapid increase in head circumference or an unusually disproportionate head shape. An abnormal shape of head may suggest underlying cause. Occipital prominence can be seen in Dandy walker malformation, whereas frontal bossing is common with aqueductal stenosis. Sutures may be splayed, and scalp veins may be very prominent.

The "setting sun" sign is an ocular abnormality where the eyes appear to look downward such that the sclera is visible above the irises. It is also known as upward gaze palsy, which usually occurs as a result of increasing pressure on region of suprapineal recess. Papilledema is a rare finding; however, long-standing hydrocephalus can lead to optic atrophy affecting vision. Motor spasticity with hyperreflexia and clonus may be present and will be more prominent in the lower extremities.

This is due to increased stretching of the motor fibers of the lower extremities as they traverse longer pathways [5]. It is important to note that if the onset of hydrocephalus is acute, then vomiting, lethargy, seizures, and cardiorespiratory compromise may occur in infants despite open sutures. In older infants, pressure on the brainstem may lead to pseudobulbar palsy where poor oral-motor control is manifest by difficulty with swallowing and changes in speech [5].

In addition, signs of growth retardation and delayed neurological development are also common. Head and trunk control is particularly affected [6].

In older children with hydrocephalus, focal neurologic signs will be more apparent. After closure of cranial sutures, older children may not have enlarged head circumference, however they tend to present with more classic signs of increased intracranial pressure such as headache and vomiting that is worse in the morning. Papilledema and abducent nerve palsy are also common findings. Clinical features can be subtle in other group of older children who have pre-existing, progressive hydrocephalus.

However, signs of psychomotor retardation or abnormal hypothalamic function such as growth derangements, delay sexual maturity, fluid and electrolyte disturbances, and thyroid dysfunction may rise the suspicion of unrecognized hydrocephalus [7,8].

Table 2. Signs and Symptoms of Pediatric Hydrocephalus

In infant and young child:
• Irritability • Impaired level of consciousness • Vomiting • Failure to thrive • Poor feeding • Developmental delay • Increasing head circumference • Poor head control • Tense anterior fontanelle • Dilated scalp veins • "Setting sun" sign (combination of upper eyelid retraction and failure of upgaze) • Bradycardia • Apnoeic spells • Seizures
In older child or adolescent: • Headache • Vomiting • Drowsiness or impaired consciousness and coma • Diplopia • Worsened seizure control • Impaired upgaze • Papilloedema

DIAGNOSIS

Most of hydrocephalus can be diagnosed through clinical evaluation. Nowadays, the diagnosis of hydrocephalus is made more readily apparent with the increasing availability of imaging techniques. Ultrasonography is useful in neonates with an open anterior fontanelle as it allows the diagnosis of ventriculomegaly at the Bedside. It also provides early detection of hydrocephalus in fetus during routine antenatal screen. In older infants and children, computed tomography (CT) may be utilized. It has a major role in accurate assessment of ventricular size, presence of hemorrhage, and location of lesion or obstruction. However, magnetic resonance imaging (MRI) is the preferred diagnostic tool in this age group as it provides less radiation and superior resolution of the brain, spinal cord, and ventricles such that specific lesions or structure abnormalities are more easily detected [9].

MANAGEMENT

Medical treatment for pediatric hydrocephalus usually is not adequate in the long term. Mannitol can be used for cases of rapidly progressive hydrocephalus, whereas medication such as acetazolamide or frusemide that decrease the production of CSF may be useful in providing temporary relief for slowly progressive hydrocephalus whilst awaiting for surgery [10,11]. In the preterm baby who has IVH, tapping of CSF is commonly performed. Repeated CSF taps (either ventricular or LP) may provide a temporizing measure until reabsorption resumes [12]. However, if spontaneous CSF resorption dose not occur, then permanent shunt will usually be necessary.

Hydrocephalus still remains a surgical condition in that the definitive treatment involves diversion of CSF into other body spaces that allows for absorption of the ventricular fluid and adequate ventricular decompression. Ventriculo-peritoneal (VP) shunting is by far the most common procedure for CSF diversion. This is achieved by the implantation of a one-way flow valve device and a permanent tube that is inserted into the lateral ventricle of the brain via a burr hole and tunneled subcutaneously into the peritoneum. Other approaches such as ventriculo-atrial (lateral ventricle to internal jugular vein), ventriculo-pleural (lateral ventricle to pleural space), and lumbo-peritoneal (lumbar intradural space to peritoneum) may be utilized as alternatives in patients who are unable to have abdominal distal catheters (e.g. multiple abdominal surgeries, recent abdominal sepsis, or known malabsorptive peritoneal cavity).

In recent years the development of adjustable shunt on the market has certainly provided another interesting dimension in the management of hydrocephalus. These programmable valves allow neurosurgeons to change valve-opening pressure or flow characteristics using an external magnetic device. The concept behind this is that CSF flow dynamics may change as the child grows, and the use of programmable shunt can allow adjustment in CSF flow without needing to perform shunt revision surgery. However recent research data has failed to demonstrate the superiority of programmable shunt over other non-adjustable shunts for its long-term benefit [11,13].

Like many other implanted devices, shunts are prone to malfunction and infection with an overall failure rate as high as 40% within the first year [11,14,15]. Causes of shunt failure can be misplacement of catheter tip, disconnection of the tubing system, over-drainage, infection, or blockage. The most common clinical findings at the time of shunt malfunction are signs and symptoms of raised ICP, which can be reliably diagnosed with CT scan and shunt series X-ray. Shunt tap may be performed if surgical exploration is considered or if infection is strongly suspected.

Recent advance of endoscopic third ventriculostomy has emerged as an alternative approach in treatment of hydrocephalus. Third ventriculostomy creates an outlet in the floor of the third ventricle that allows CSF to escape into the basal cistern so that it can circulate in the extracerebral subarachnoid space and to be absorbed. The ideal patient for this procedure is the older child who has obstruction at the level of the aqueduct of Sylvius. However, the success rate in infant may be poor because they may not have a normally developed subarachnoid space. In addition, third ventriculostomy has also been proposed as a treatment option for patients who developed over-shunting (e.g. subdural hematomas, slit ventricle syndrome) after insertion of CSF flow diversion shunt. Previously, third ventriculostomy has been attempted in many other types of hydrocephalus but appears less successful in communicating hydrocephalus such as post-hemorrhagic and post-meningitis.

PROGNOSIS AND OUTCOME

Pediatric hydrocephalus is usually a lifelong disorder. The overall outcome and prognosis of hydrocephalus is highly dependent on multiple factors including the age of onset, underlying etiology, duration and extent of neurologic damage prior to correction of the intracranial insult, as well as response to treatment. Despite the significant decrease in mortality following shunt placement, there is still much long-term morbidity associated with the disorder [16]. How a pediatric patient functions in society is perhaps the ultimate measure of outcome. The important functional concerns usually include impaired mobility, impaired cognition, sensory deficits, endocrine dysfunction (e.g. growth, weight balance, fertility, and puberty), epilepsy, depression, and pain. Regardless the present data suggesting the frequency of these potential debilitating sequelae, early diagnosis and treatment of hydrocephalus will be the key to prevent associated morbidity and mortality [17]. As for neurosurgeons, their undisputed role is to avoid post-operative complication. Last but not least, multidisciplinary planning and close follow-up is needed to ensure the maximal developmental potential of these children.

References

[1] Del Bigio MR. Neuropathology and structural changes in hydrocephalus. *Developmental disabilities research reviews,* 2010;16(1):16-22.

[2] James HE. Hydrocephalus in infancy and childhood. *American family physician,* Feb 1992;45(2):733-742.

[3] Partington MD. Congenital hydrocephalus. *Neurosurgery clinics of North America,* Oct 2001;12(4):737-742, ix.

[4] van de Bor M, Verloove-Vanhorick SP, Brand R, Keirse MJ, Ruys JH. Incidence and prediction of periventricular-intraventricular hemorrhage in very preterm infants. *Journal of perinatal medicine,* 1987;15(4):333-339.

[5] Fishman MA. Developmental Defects. In: McMillan JA DC, Feigin RD, Warshaw JB, ed. Oski's Pediatrics: Principles and Practice. 3rd ed. Philadelphia: Lippincott Williams and Wilkins; 1999:1906-1909.

[6] Rizvi R, Anjum Q. Hydrocephalus in children. *JPMA. The Journal of the Pakistan Medical Association,* Nov 2005;55(11):502-507.

[7] Shallat RF, Pawl RP, Jerva MJ. Significance of upward gaze palsy (Parinaud's syndrome) in hydrocephalus due to shunt malfunction. *Journal of neurosurgery,* Jun 1973;38(6):717-721.

[8] Merchant TE, Lee H, Zhu J, et al. The effects of hydrocephalus on intelligence quotient in children with localized infratentorial ependymoma before and after focal radiation therapy. *Journal of neurosurgery,* Nov 2004;101(2 Suppl):159-168.

[9] Bradley WG, Jr. Diagnostic tools in hydrocephalus. *Neurosurgery clinics of North America,* Oct 2001;12(4):661-684, viii.

[10] Kanev PM, Park TS. The treatment of hydrocephalus. *Neurosurgery clinics of North America,* Oct 1993;4(4):611-619.

[11] Kestle JR. Pediatric hydrocephalus: current management. *Neurologic clinics,* Nov 2003;21(4):883-895, vii.

[12] Kreusser KL, Tarby TJ, Kovnar E, Taylor DA, Hill A, Volpe JJ. Serial lumbar punctures for at least temporary amelioration of neonatal posthemorrhagic hydrocephalus. *Pediatrics,* Apr 1985;75(4):719-724.

[13] Pollack IF, Albright AL, Adelson PD. A randomized, controlled study of a programmable shunt valve versus a conventional valve for patients with hydrocephalus. Hakim-Medos Investigator Group. *Neurosurgery,* Dec 1999;45(6):1399-1408; discussion 1408-1311.

[14] Lo P, Drake JM. Shunt malfunctions. *Neurosurgery clinics of North America,* Oct 2001;12(4):695-701, viii.

[15] Drake JM, Kestle JT. Determining the best cerebrospinal fluid shunt valve design: the pediatric valve design trial. *Neurosurgery,* Nov 1998;43(5):1259-1260.

[16] Hoppe-Hirsch E, Laroussinie F, Brunet L, et al. Late outcome of the surgical treatment of hydrocephalus. *Child's nervous system : ChNS : official journal of the International Society for Pediatric Neurosurgery,* Mar 1998;14(3):97-99.

[17] Vinchon M, Rekate HL, Kulkarni AV. Pediatric hydrocephalus outcomes: a review. *Fluids and barriers of the CNS,* Aug 27 2012;9(1):18.

In: Hydrocephalus
Editor: Amaya Velazquez
ISBN: 978-1-62100-453-0

Chapter 5

HEMORRHAGIC HYDROCEPHALUS (*HHY*): A NOVEL HYDROCEPHALUS MOUSE MUTATION WITH NEAR-PERFECT PENETRANCE

***Nobuko Mori*[1], *Mitsuru Kuwamura*[2] *and Natsuki Tanaka*[2]**

[1]Department of Biological Science, Graduate School of Science, Osaka Prefecture University, Naka-ku, Sakai-shi, Japan

[2]Division of Veterinary Medicine, Graduate School of Life and Environmental Sciences, Osaka Prefecture University, Izumisano-shi, Osaka, Japan

ABSTRACT

Genetic factors play a role in the development of human hydrocephalus. However, little is known about the pathogenesis of human congenital hydrocephalus. Recently, we identified coiled-coil domain-containing 85C (*Ccdc85c*) as a causative gene for hemorrhagic hydrocephalus (*hhy*) mouse mutation exhibiting an autosomally recessive pattern of inheritance. Mice homozygous for *hhy* develop communicating hydrocephalus at near-perfect penetrance, with heads bulged from accumulating cerebrospinal fluid within several days after birth. These mice exhibit a variational ventricular dilatation with frequent brain hemorrhage at biopsy and also develop subcortical band heterotopia, a malformation of cerebral cortex in all cases. Furthermore, these mutant mice showed agenesis of the ependymal layer lining the cerebral cortex, a possible cause of hydrocephalus. Analyses of corticogenesis at embryonic days revealed that premature depletion of cortical radial glia, neural progenitors performing both embryonal neurogenesis and postnatal gliogenesis, underlay the *hhy* phenotype. The *hh*y mutant may be a useful animal model in understanding the pathogenesis of hydrocephalus.

INTRODUCTION

Hydrocephalus is a common medical condition ascribable to abnormalities in the production, flow or resorption of cerebrospinal fluid (CSF). Accumulation of CSF in the ventricular system results in ventricular dilatation, a major criterion for hydrocephalus in clinical diagnosis, and cerebral dysfunction. Human hydrocephalus is classified into two classes: congenital and acquired. Congenital hydrocephalus cases are frequently accompanied by complication of developmental abnormalities, mostly considered to be heritable. However, causative genes and pathogenesis of human congenital hydrocephalus have been poorly understood [1].

Genetic and pathological analysis of hydrocephalus mutations using animal models might be helpful in understanding mechanisms underlying pathogenesis and also in the development of effective treatment of the disease. In this chapter, we discuss genetics and pathogenesis of hemorrhagic hydrocephalus (*hhy*) mouse mutation, which we recently identified in coiled-coil domain-containing 85c (*Ccdc85c*) [2, 3], in comparison with other hydrocephalus mutants.

Development of Communicating Hydrocephalus with Near-Perfect Penetrance in *hhy* Mice

The autosomal recessive hemorrhagic hydrocephalus *hhy* mutation occurred spontaneously in the colony of a congenic strain of mice carrying a portion of STS-derived chromosome 4 in the BALB/cHeA (BALB/c) background at the animal facility of the Osaka prefecture university. The clinical manifestation of the disease is characterized with an expanded cranium due to accumulation of CSF in the ventricular cavities in the *hhy* mutants (Figure 1).

Mostly, it becomes obvious within two weeks after birth. Because neither stenosis nor obstruction was detected in the ventricular system of affected animals, hydrocephalus in the *hhy* mutant was classified into a communicating type. In many cases affected with hydrocephalus, intracranial hemorrhage was observed. Intriguingly, bleeding was not detected in any other organs, hence being confined to the brain. All of the mutants examined had heterotopia in the white matter, while cortical lamination of the mutants was largely normal. Band-like distribution of heterotopia under the normal lamination of the *hhy* cortex is reminiscent of the human X-linked doublecortin (DCX) mutation, the causative gene of which is involved in microtubule stabilization [4]. Therefore, we hypothesized that the *hhy* mutation might impinge on neuronal migration in the developing cerebrum. Although intractable epilepsy has been associated with heterotopia in humans [5], the *hhy* mutants have hitherto not exhibited epileptic seizure. Except for subcortical heterotopia, neither morphological nor vascular anomaly was observed in the *hhy* brain. After mapping the *hhy* mutation to chromosome 12, mice heterozygous for the BALB/c-derived chromosomal segment containing the *hhy* mutation was backcrossed to MSM/Ms (MSM) mice, and the heterozygous *hhy* mutant allele was maintained in the MSM background. In the course of fine mapping, we examined 256 animals including recombinants and their offspring.

Among them, 29 animals clinically affected with hydrocephalus were homozygous for the BALB/c allele in the region critical for the *hhy* mutation; the remaining 227 unaffected animals had BALB/c and MSM heterozygous or MSM homozygous allele in the *hhy* region. Thus, the *hhy* mutation develops a communicating type of ydrocephalus with near-perfect penetrance, without showing any developmental abnormalities in the brain except for subcortical heterotopia.

Premature Depletion of Nascent Neural Progenitor Radial Glial Cells Underlies the Mechanism for Hydrocephalus as Well as Heterotopia in *hhy* Mice

Cortical radial glial cells (RGCs) are highly polarized neural progenitors residing on the ventricular wall surface in the developing cortex, extending long radial fibers anchoring the basal lamina, i.e., pia mater, and protruding short apical projections called apical endfeet into the lateral ventricles filled with CSF. RGCs are multipotent progenitors capable of differentiating into neurons and glial cells such as astroglial cells, oligodendrocytes and ependymal cells lining the ventricular wall surface in the mature brain. RGCs perform interkinetic nuclear migration synchronized with cell cycling within the ventricular zone (VZ): they perform DNA synthesis at the border between the VZ and subventricular zone (SVZ) and planer cell divisions on the ventricular wall surface [6, 7]. During the nuclear movement, apicobasal polarity of RGCs is maintained by the adherens junctions connecting their apical end feet to each other, which exhibit circumferential rings of junctional molecules on the ventricular wall surface. Thus, proliferating RGCs produce basal progenitors, i.e., progenitors committed to neurons with limited proliferation ability and concomitantly self-renew during cortical development in the embryonic days. After birth, however, RGCs are drastically eliminated from the VZ, turning, in part, into ciliated ependymal cells lining the ventricular wall surface. Nascent ependymal cell progenitors are RGCs, mostly born during embryonic (E) day 14 (E14)–E16, the later stage of neurogenesis [8].

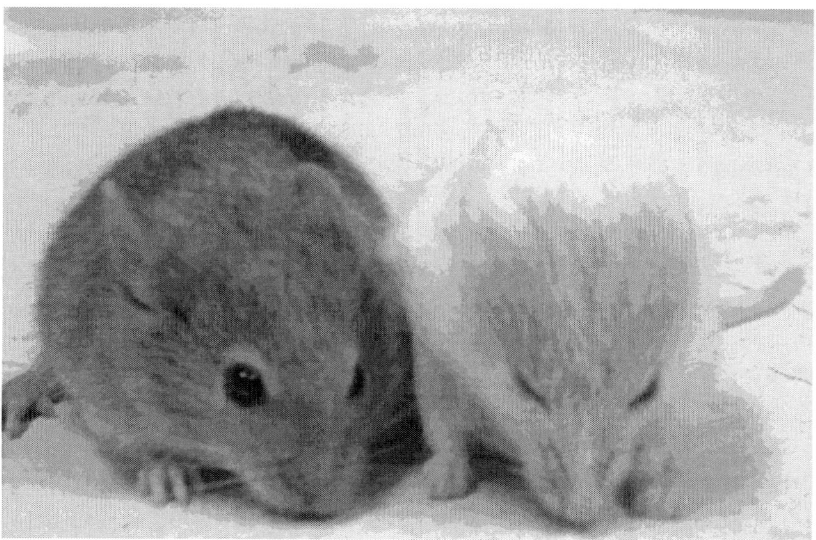

Figure 1. The *hhy* mouse affected with hydrocephalus. The *hhy* mutant at two weeks (Right) and an age-matched control (Left). The *hhy* mutant has a dome-shaped head caused by accumulation of CSF and the black face due to intracranial hemorrhage.

The *hhy* mice develop a communicating type of hydrocephalus. The mutants lacked ciliated ependymal cells on the dorsal surface of the lateral ventricular walls with bare neuroblasts in direct contact with CSF at birth (3).

As indicated by the presence of phagocytes, inflammatory response occurred on the ventricular wall surface in the neonatal *hhy* mutants. Radial fibers as well as somas of RGCs positively stained with nestin, a neuroepithelial-specific intermediate filament protein, were largely eliminated in the mutant at E18, and instead heterotopic cells were widely distributed in the subcortical zone. Cells in the subcortical heterotopia of the *hhy* brain were positively stained with special AT-rich sequence binding protein 2 (Satb2), a marker of neurons in the upper cortical layers II–IV containing neurons born at E15–E16. BrdU-labeling experiments also demonstrated that cells in the subcortical heterotopia of the *hhy* brain were born at the later stage of neurogenesis. Our data indicate that *hhy* mice have an abnormality in RGCs as nascent progenitors for ependymal cells and as a scaffold for neuronal migration. RGCs expressing a transcription factor paired box gene 6 (Pax6) are normally concentrated within the VZ [9]. Basal progenitors born to RGCs by planer division on the ventricular wall surface express a transcription factor T-box brain protein 2 (Tbr2) instead of Pax6, changing their position from VZ to the SVZ in the developing cortex. Hence, a laminated structure of the VZ and SVZ can be visualized by stain for Pax6 and Tbr2. Post-mitotic neurons in the cortical plate and in the intermediate zone between the SVZ and the cortex are positively stained with T-box brain protein 1 (Tbr1). In the *hhy* brain, dislocation of a considerable part of proliferating Pax6-positive cells outside of their normal residence VZ occurred at E14, at which lamination of the Tbr2-positive cells was normal. At advanced stage of neurogenesis, however, not only Pax6-positive cells but also Tbr2-positive cells were massively dislocated from their intrinsic niches VZ and SVZ to the entire subcortical region of the *hhy* brain at E16, thereby abolishing the laminated structure. Pax6-positive cells were almost entirely eliminated from the VZ of the *hhy* brain at E18. On the other hand, Tbr1-positive neurons, progeny of early-born basal progenitors, were properly layered in the developing cortical plate of the *hhy* embryo. Taken together, RGCs on the ventricular wall surface were prematurely depleted through basal dislocation in the *hhy* brain. Hence, both ependymal agenesis at birth and migration failure, at least in part, of later-born neurons in the *hhy* brain are explained by abnormal behavior of RGCs during neurogenesis.

Defective Ependyma is a Validated Cause for Communicating Hydrocephalus in Mice

Ciliated ependymal cells are almost certainly important during brain development. Ciliary dysgenesis and/or dysfunction result in communicating type of hydrocephalus in several mouse mutants. Some mutations are implicated in defects in ciliary motility: *Hydin* in autosomal recessive hydrocephalus-3 (*hy-3*), *Spag6* in sperm-associated antigen 6 (*Spag6*) and dynein, axonemal, heavy chain 5 (*Dnahc5*) are all ciliary axoneme-associated proteins, deficiency of which causes dyskinesia of ependymal cilia, resulting in defective fluid-clearance and accumulation of CSF in the brain ventricles, i.e., hydrocephalus [10–12]. A defect in intraflagellar transport 88 homolog (*ift88*)/polaris/Tg737 also causes communicating type of hydrocephalus [13]. Ift88, a component of an IFT particle, is indispensable for ciliary assembly. In addition, recent investigation showed that planar cell polarity-signaling proteins Celsr2 and Celsr3 are involved in ependymal cilia development and in the pathophysiology of hydrocephalus [14]. Although these causative genes for hydrocephalus have a variety of subcellular functions, all of the defective mutations in these genes result in a simple pathological mechanism, i.e., ciliary abnormality that results in impaired CSF flow.

A mutation in N-ethylmaleimide sensitive fusion protein attachment protein alpha (*Napa*) encoding αSNAP is causative for autosomal recessive hydrocephaly with hop gate (*hyh*) [15]. The *hyh* mutant develops communicating hydrocephalus within embryonic days and dies after birth from progressive enlargement of the ventricular system, which is induced by stenosis of the aqueduct generated after birth [16]. The *hyh* mutant has a markedly small cortex, exhibiting defective neurogenesis. The SVZ in postnatal *hyh* mice is morphologically disrupted with a marked reduction of proliferative cells in the stem cell niche [17]. The *hyh* mice had severely disrupted ependymal layer and nodular heterotopia along the denuded ventricular wall [18)]. The data suggest a defect in RGCs in the *hyh* mutant, similar to the *hhy* case. However, pathophysiology of hydrocephalus in the *hyh* mutant appears to be complicated. Because αSNAP is critical for recycling SNARE proteins that tether vesicles to membrane in membrane traffic, defective exocytosis may affect a broad spectrum of physiological and developmental pathways. Although subcellular functions of the Ccdc85C protein remain to be elucidated, Ccdc85C may control self-renewal of RGCs through signaling from apical junctions during cortical neurogenesis.

Conclusion

Hydrocephalus in the *hhy* mutant is due to premature depletion of RGCs leading to ependymal agenesis. Our study showed a novel mechanism for a communicating type of hydrocephalus with near-perfect penetrance in the *hhy* mutant, providing a useful animal model in understanding pathogenesis of hydrocephalus in humans.

References

[1] Zang J, Williams MA, Rigmonti D, Genetics of human hydrocephalus. *J. Neurol.* 253: 1255–1266, 2006.

[2] Kuwamura M, Kinoshita A, Okumoto M, Yamate J, Mori N, Hemorrhagic hydrocephalus (*hhy*): a novel mutation on mouse chromosome 12. *Brain Res. Dev. Brain Res.* 152: 69–72, 2004.

[3] Mori N, Kuwamura M, Tanaka N, Hirano R, Nabe M, Ibuki M, Yamate J, *Ccdc85c* encoding a protein at the apical junctions of radial glia is disrupted in hemorrhagic hydrocephalus (*hhy*) mice. *Am. J. Pathol.* 180: 314–327, 2012.

[4] Caspi M, Atlas R, Kantor A, Sapir T, Reiner O, Interaction between LIS1 and doublecortin, two lissencephaly gene products. *Hum. Mol. Genet.* 9:2205-2213, 2000.

[5] Rang T, Atefy R, Sheen V, Malformation of cortical development. *Neurologist* 14: 181–191, 2008.

[6] Anthony TE, Klein C, Fishell G, Heintz N, Radial glia serve as neuronal progenitors in all regions of the central nervous system. *Neuron.* 41:881–890, 2004.

[7] Noctor SC, Martínez-Cerdeño V, Ivic L, Kriegstein AR, Cortical neurons arise in symmetric and asymmetric division zones and migrate through specific phases. *Nat. Neurosci.* 7:136-144, 2004.

[8] Spassky N, Merkle FT, Flames N, Tramontin AD, García-Verdugo JM, Alvarez-Buylla A, Adult ependymal cells are postmitotic and are derived

from radial glial cells during embryogenesis. *J. Neurosci.* 25:10-18, 2005.

[9] Englund C, Fink A, Lau C, Pham D, Daza RA, Bulfone A, Kowalczyk T, Hevner RF, Pax6, Tbr2, and Tbr1 are expressed sequentially by radial glia, intermediate progenitor cells, and postmitotic neurons in developing neocortex. *J. Neurosci.* 25:247-251, 2005.

[10] Davy BE, Robinson ML, Congenital hydrocephalus in *hy3* mice is caused by a frameshift mutation in *Hydin*, a large novel gene. *Hum Mol Genet* 12:1163-1170, 2003.

[11] Sapiro R, Kostetskii I, Olds-Clarke P, Gerton GL, Radice GL, Strauss JF III. Male infertility, impaired sperm motility, and hydrocephalus in mice deficient in sperm-associated antigen 6. *Mol. Cell Biol.* 22: 6298-6305, 2002.

[12] Ibañez-Tallon I, Gorokhova S, Heintz N. Loss of function of axonemal dynein Mdnah5 causes primary ciliary dyskinesia and hydrocephalus. *Hum. Mol. Genet.* 11:715-721, 2002.

[13] Taulman PD, Haycraft CJ, Balkovetz DF, Yoder BK, Polaris, a protein involved in left-right axis patterning, localizes to basal bodies and cilia. *Mol. Biol. Cell* 12:589-599, 2001.

[14] Tissir F, Qu Y, Montcouquiol M, Zhou L, Komatsu K, Shi D, Fujimori T, Labeau J, Tyteca D, Courtoy P, Poumay Y, Uemura T, Goffinet AM, Lack of cadherins Celsr2 and Celsr3 impairs ependymal ciliogenesis, leading to fatal hydrocephalus. *Nature Neurosci.* 13:700–707, 2010.

[15] Chae TH, Kim S, Marz KE, Hanson PI, Walsh CA, The *hyh* mutation uncovers roles for alpha Snap in apical protein localization and control of neural cell fate. *Nat. Genet.* 36:264-270, 2004.

[16] Wagner C, Batiz LF, Rodríguez S, Jiménez AJ, Páez P, Tomé M, Pérez-Fígares JM, Rodríguez EM, Cellular mechanisms involved in the stenosis and obliteration of the cerebral aqueduct of *hyh* mutant mice developing congenital hydrocephalus. *J. Neuropathol. Exp. Neurol.* 62:1019-1040, 2003.

[17] Jiménez AJ, García-Verdugo JM, González CA, Bátiz LF, Rodríguez-Pérez LM, Páez P, Soriano-Navarro M, Roales-Buján R, Rivera P, Rodríguez S, Rodríguez EM, Pérez-Fígares JM Disruption of the neurogenic niche in the subventricular zone of postnatal hydrocephalic *hyh* mice. *J. Neuropathol. Exp. Neurol.* 68:1006-1020, 2009.

[18] Ferland RJ, Batiz LF, Neal J, Lian G, Bundock E, Lu J, Hsiao YC, Diamond R, Mei D, Banham AH, Brown PJ, Vanderburg CR, Joseph J, Hecht JL, Folkerth R, Guerrini R, Walsh CA, Rodriguez EM, Sheen VL,

Disruption of neural progenitors along the ventricular and subventricular zones in periventricular heterotopia. *Hum. Mol. Genet.* 18: 497-516, 2009.

INDEX

B

C

D

E

N

O

P

Q

R

S

T

U

V

W

Y